THE EIGHT LIMBS OF YOGA FOR MODERN TIMES

A PRACTICAL GUIDE TO THE YOGA
SUTRAS OF PATANJALI

Michelle S. Fondin

Also by Michelle S. Fondin

The Empowered Divine Feminine: Becoming an Unstoppable Woman in the 21st Century and Beyond

Twin Flame Union: 7 Keys to a Healthy Twin Flame Journey

Heal Yourself A Return to Wholeness: The Integration of Body, Mind, Soul, and Spirit

Twin Flame Romance: The Journey to Unconditional Love

Chakra Healing for Vibrant Energy: Exploring Your 7 Energy Centers with Mindfulness, Yoga, and Ayurveda

Enlightened Medicine Your Power to Get Well Now: An Integrative Approach to Healing the Seven Deadly Lifestyle Diseases

Help! I Think My Loved One Is an Alcoholic: A Survival Guide for Lovers, Family, and Friends

How to Run a Yoga Business and Not Go Broke: Lessons from a Yoga Teacher, Entrepreneur, and Modern Hippie

The Wheel of Healing with Ayurveda: An Easy Guide to a Healthy Lifestyle

The Wheel of Healing with Ayurveda Companion Workbook

Forbidden Fruit: An Unlikely Love Story

Contents

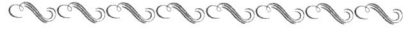

Wake up from this dream of separateness.

The Shevatashvatara Upanishad

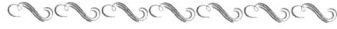

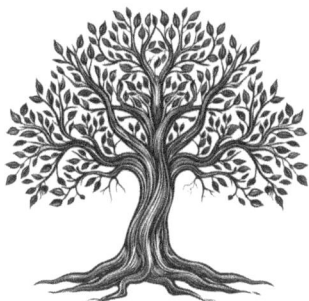

Preface

I will never forget my first yoga class. I sat on the hardwood floor of the community center in West Bloomfield, Michigan with eager anticipation. The excitement I felt had little to do with learning yoga and everything to do with the environment. The year was 1989. I had just graduated from high school, and my boyfriend Chris, who was eight years my senior, had urged me to sign up for an eight-week yoga session taught by my high school religion teacher. While I had little interest in yoga, I was excited to spend time with my boyfriend. Little did I know my life would be forever transformed over the next ninety minutes.

The community center room was already filled with students when we arrived. It was so crowded we had to place our beach towels at the front of the class. Most of the students seemed well-versed in yoga. They were stretching or doing headstands while I stared in amazement. Finally, my former school teacher, Lee Ann, entered the room. Sprite and energetic, Lee Ann saw us immediately and guided us closer to the front. Even with her four feet eleven-inch stature, she commanded the room. Throughout the class, I fell into a pleasurable, trance-like state I couldn't explain. Exercise wasn't foreign to me. I had been taking group fitness classes since I was twelve and grew up in the world of classical ballet. But this was different, something I couldn't quite define. Lee Ann's voice and guidance lit up a part of me that radiated stronger than a beacon guiding a ship at night. After ninety minutes, I was hooked.

While I experienced yoga on and off during my twenties and early thirties, it wasn't until my yoga teacher training in 2007 that I began to understand my all-encompassing comfort in practicing yoga. Yoga spoke to me, not as an exercise program but as something profound and expansive. The broad scope of my feelings began to unfold as I learned about the Yoga Sutras of Patanjali. I then understood that yoga asana only reflects a small part of a broader philosophy and lifestyle.

While Chris and I experienced our first yoga classes together, I discovered that his role in my life had always been that of an off-the-mat yoga teacher.

Below, you'll discover the reasons why.

According to the Eight Limbs of Yoga, as expressed by Patanjali, yoga is a way of life. It's a philosophy that leads you to union with yourself. Chris unknowingly taught me many yogic principles before our first mat class together. He presented me with books on yoga philosophy, Zen Buddhism, mindfulness (dharana), and meditation (dhyana). Through the Kama Sutra, he taught me the practice of spiritual love-making (brahmacharya). He followed a vegetarian diet and encouraged me to do the same (ahimsa). He read me stories about present-moment awareness and non-attachment (aparigraha) by Richard and Leslie Bach. And even though I didn't understand it then, he loved me unconditionally by letting me explore my path as I ventured off to college.

Before I tasted the delight of my first asana practice, I was primed, pumped, and ready with the lessons Chris had taught me about living a yogic lifestyle.

While a physical yoga practice has been a part of my life for over thirty-five years, living a yoga lifestyle is my daily practice.

In 2008, I earned my certifications to teach yoga, meditation, and an Ayurvedic lifestyle through the Chopra Center. I then opened my yoga center, The Ayurvedic Path, and taught thousands of students over ten years. Even though I loved teaching, I felt my students were missing something: *the eagerness for a deeper spiritual understanding.*

Most came to my studio for physical or emotional relief. My students wanted to get fit, reduce stress, or become healthier, all worthwhile goals. However, they only sought band-aid fixes for their deeper problems. They felt fine if they took a class. But returned to square one if they missed a few weeks. You probably know the feeling if you've had a regular gym routine and then missed a month or two. After returning, the soreness in your muscles told you how much you slacked off.

Since yoga is an integrative practice, even a simple asana practice does much more than the eye can see. That is what I wanted my students to understand. When you grasp the true meaning of yoga as a philosophy, you can choose to never do another yoga posture and still reach enlightenment.

Many gifts lie in the container of the Yoga Sutras that move you toward wholeness. I invite you to open the boxes containing the Eight Limbs of Yoga, then explore and analyze each to see if they speak to you. I have found them delicious and inviting as I move along my life path. The Yoga Sutras are ageless and timeless principles for living more holistically. I aim to pull these yoga principles into modern times to make them useful and relevant.

With the popularity of yoga in the Western world today, I am compelled to share the fullness of the Eight Limbs of Yoga with those who only know yoga asana. Intuitively, most of us feel this holistic pull when we take a yoga class. That might be one of the reasons yoga has grown by leaps and bounds over the past twenty years. For those who start yoga for the physical effects but continue to gain more, learning about the spiritual aspects can be helpful. For some, the vanity of yoga and its enormous merchandising push can cause them to lose sight of the subtleties of yoga's capacity to heal and create amazing human beings.

I share this vision to allow for holistic growth on all levels. In our goal-oriented Western mindset, we often lose sight of the process. The goal of yoga is the process. Even perfecting a yoga asana is not the end goal. Whether we've been practicing for three days or thirty years, we are all in the process of becoming. As in all instances of spiritual evolution, the result always leads to a new beginning. We are never finished until we take our last breath, and even then...

Perhaps you came to this book because it's required for your yoga teacher training. Or, maybe you want to deepen your yoga asana practice or are curious about Eastern philosophy. Whatever your reasons, they are valid. I hope to make this journey into the Yoga Sutras fun, compelling, light, and easy to understand.

Before we begin, I'd like to comment on the use of Sanskrit terms. The Yoga Sutras, like most ancient Indian texts, were written in Sanskrit. Having studied Sanskrit with my teacher, Dr. David Simon, I thought about including the Sutras in Sanskrit and English but decided against it. Upon reading several translations, I found that muddling my way through a hybrid Sanskrit/ English text was disruptive. I want the reading experience to be as smooth as possible; to that end, I've sprinkled in Sanskrit terms with their English translation the first time the term is mentioned. Additionally, you will find a glossary of Sanskrit terms at the end of the book.

Finally, the Yoga Sutras mentioned are only a fraction of the 196 verses. Most of the verses pertaining to the Eight Limbs of Yoga are from Part 2 of the Yoga Sutras, and you will find the exact verse to refer to at the end of each quote. For further reading of the complete Yoga Sutras, please refer to the Bibliography.

I urge you to study the Eight Limbs of Yoga with the ever-present innocence I had when taking my first yoga class: expect nothing and gain everything. Stay open and willing, and you will have a magical spiritual journey. Let's go! *Hari om tat sat* (I am that. You are that. All this is that.)

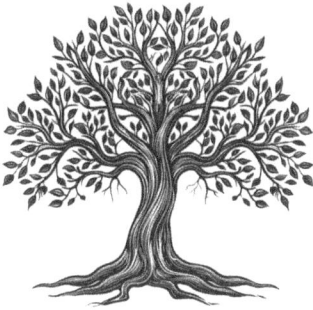

Introduction

The Yoga Sutras and The Eight Limbs of Yoga

The Self is one, though it appears to be many. Those who meditate upon the Self and realize the Self go beyond decay and death, beyond separateness and sorrow. They see the Self in everyone and obtain all things.
- 26.2 The Chandogya Upanishad

The Yoga Sutras are the pathway to self-realization. But what is this *Self*? And what does it have to do with yoga?
The answer is— Everything.

In modern times, upon hearing self-realization, one might think of the words selfish, self-centered, or selfie, all indicating a preoccupation with oneself. And yet, while self-centeredness has its place in enlightenment, the "Self" is the higher self or Spirit. Since yoga means "to yoke" or "unite," your yoga practice unites your body, mind, emotions, soul, and higher self or Spirit. Therefore, self-realization is the inward journey toward uniting every part of you, leading to enlightenment. The meaning of this will unfold as you learn about the Eight Limbs of Yoga.

The Yoga Sutras of Patanjali

The Vedas are well-known books of knowledge from the Indus River valley in what is now known as India. The Vedic texts, The Upanishads, are said to have been passed down from teacher to student anywhere between 2,000 to 2,500 years BCE. At the time, the Vedas were an oral tradition taught through poetry and song. By the time Patanjali (either one person or a group of persons) formed the 196 verses to become the Yoga Sutras, Vedic thought had barely begun to be written. It is said that the Yoga Sutras were formed anywhere between 200 years BCE and 400 CE. Patanjali formed the Yoga Sutras directly from *The Upanishads*, most notably the *Rig Veda*. The Eight Limbs of Yoga were extracted from these Yoga Sutras around 600 CE and applied to a classical yoga practice called *Ashtanga*, or eight limbs. These are the Yoga Sutras I will outline in this book.

Many interpreters of the Yoga Sutras, including B.K.S. Iyengar, Swami Kriyananda, and Sri Swami Satchidananda, claim that yoga philosophy transcends religion. Yet, upon reading their translations and others, I found that these men, disciplined in their studies, explained yoga very much like a set of strict rules that one must follow to attain self-realization. It appears that the more they studied and applied the dogma of the Yoga Sutra practices, the more religious they became. I'm offering a more refreshing approach.

In studying The Upanishads, the inspiration of the verses transcended the words on the pages. In other words, the essence throughout the stories and poems of The Upanishads feels like a song to Brahma or the Lord. It doesn't feel like religious dogma when reading it. Instead, it feels exhilarating. And yet, once seasoned gurus translated it into a strict lifestyle, it became devoid of its magic. That said, I don't think that was the intention of the scholars who interpreted the Yoga Sutras. Turning the spiritual into something functional is a byproduct of human nature. We want order and a system in societies, schools, and ashrams. But the system takes over, leaving inspiration by the wayside.

The Yoga Sutras are guides like the guardrails in a bowling lane. They're wise and filled with ancient traditions to help you on your yogic path. The map that the Yoga Sutras provide is not the experience itself. Once you can reach transcendence and union with the Divine, you no longer need the map. You will always feel compelled toward the right action. Therefore, the Yoga Sutras exist for you to follow until you no longer need them.

Additionally, we mustn't use the Yoga Sutras to assess good or bad and right or wrong. Many previous interpreters wrote much about the rightness and wrongness of behavior. Pure spirit is unconditional love. And unconditional love is free from judgment about right and wrong. Just as there are many ways to conduct a business or get through school, many paths can lead you to the same outcome. And you don't have to shun your human nature to get there.

Discipline is the value you need to get you to your destination. If the Eight Limbs of Yoga speak to you as they spoke to me, allow them to give you the discipline, strength, and guidance to get to the place within yourself that will lead you to your Divine destiny.

Written By Men for Men

Upanishad translates to "sitting at the feet of" a spiritual teacher or guru. In the Indus River valley, young men would move to forest academies to sit with their gurus for an average of twelve years until they reached enlightenment. Afterward, many would return to their villages to marry and live their lives as householders. To this day, The Upanishads remain, by far, among the most essential Vedic texts for Hindus.

The word *sutra* means "suture" or "to thread." The eight-limbed path of the Yoga Sutras works to thread together the aspects of the Self toward wholeness. As mentioned in the previous section, these practices help the practitioner point toward one common goal.

However, one thing to remember while studying the Yoga Sutras is that the Vedic texts and Yoga Sutras were written by men for men. It's important to note this as some wording can seem like harsh religious rhetoric or outdated patriarchal views. As an interpreter of the Eight Limbs of Yoga, I'd like you to see them for what they are, not how they're worded.

Before modern times, spiritual teachers got young men, as young as eleven or twelve, and had to keep them on the straight and narrow for many years until adulthood. Hundreds, if not thousands, lived in these forest academies to learn the pathway to enlightenment. And yet, they were boys like any other boys. They were growing with hormones and normal boyhood curiosities. Like a modern-day school, the teachers had to keep them attentive and on task.

If we were to extract words from the Yoga Sutras verbatim and apply them to our modern life, much of it wouldn't make sense. According to an article in The Washington Post in 2024, out of the 34 million Americans practicing yoga, twice the number of women to men take yoga classes.[1] This statistic is the polar opposite of ancient times. The yoga practiced by men in the forest academies wasn't what we see today. Since the intent was enlightenment, the spiritual teachers taught their students to meditate for hours daily. Therefore, the Yoga Sutras were designed toward that purpose.

To that end, I encourage you to look at the Eight Limbs of Yoga as guidelines for living a fuller and healthier life rather than a dogmatic practice that must be followed to the letter.

Why Study the Eight Limbs of Yoga?

In 2025, yoga is everywhere. When I started practicing in 1989, I had to look hard to find a yoga class. Now, you can take yoga at your gym, community center, school, yoga center, or hotel when you're on vacation. If you don't want to leave the comfort of your home, you can find hundreds of thousands of yoga videos on YouTube or a yoga app. So, with yoga becoming as commonplace as walking or running, why bother studying the philosophy behind the class?

I can think of many reasons to study the Yoga Sutras and the Eight Limbs of Yoga, but here are three to start.

1. The Attainment of Stillness

The cause of most illnesses in modern times is the perception of stress and how it's received in the body. The demands of modern life far exceed what we're meant to do on our own. In many modern societies, we're expected to have two household incomes, raise children without extended families nearby, and meet the status quo by owning a home, two cars, fashionable clothing, and the latest gadgets. To be good parents and provide for our children, we must have them in the best schools, the top sports teams, and various expensive extra-curricular activities. Moreover, to be productive and good members of society, parents must volunteer and coach teams. Single parents are expected to be everything to their children to ensure the best life possible. And for those without children, societal pressures amount to having the best job, the ultimate education, and the drive to move up the corporate ladder. The mantra for today seems to be "more."

The attainment of stillness, even momentary, will help you decipher between what you want to have and achieve and what is the result of societal conditioning. External voices will no longer influence you because you will have found your authentic inner voice.

Stillness will allow you to connect with the pulse and heartbeat of the universe so you become aligned with it.

2. The Subconscious Quest for Meaning

We have more than enough information. What we're starving for is wisdom.

—-*Tony Robbins*

We live in the information age. We can search for any fact and instantaneously get the answer. Information, while valuable to some extent, doesn't give you the satisfaction of direct experience. As yogis, we're outliers. We're on a quest for deeper meaning and wisdom.

Even if you've attained what society has expected of you, you might feel that a bigger piece is missing, though you're not sure what. The Yoga Sutras offer a pathway for clearing the clutter of social conditioning to see the depth and meaning inside of you.

3. To Move from Separateness to Wholeness and from Darkness to Light

Lead me from the unreal to the Real. Lead me from darkness to light. Lead me from death to immortality.

- Brihadaranyaka Upanishad 1.3.28

When you come to the end of this section, if you understand it with every fiber of your being, you won't need to read the rest of this book.

The entire purpose of the practice and philosophy of yoga is to help you understand that you are not separate from your Source or God. In The Upanishads, God is referred to as the Self. It is also referred to as Brahman or the Lord of Life. The name is irrelevant since God cannot be confined to a name.

Through yoga, you realize that you are the Source in physical form. You came as Source energy into this physical body to experience life. Before you were born, you agreed to forget that you are indeed Source. In that agreement, you took on personal aspects, including the body, intellect, mind, ego, emotions, and individual soul. You also took on an energy and environmental body, which attaches you to your surroundings.

Because you are Source energy in physical form, you are hard-wired to search for oneness.[1] And when you attach yourself to physical things, you never feel quite whole. And that is because of the impermanent nature of the physical.

Therefore, yoga helps you remember who you are. Once you realize who you truly are, you cease to suffer, and the fear of death is gone because you know you are immortal.

In this enlightened state, you become a beacon of light for others. Once you have experiential knowledge of wholeness, you can always find it again.

In this way, the yogic path is only a path. It's a map to guide you toward your God-realized Self. That is

---

1 In this book, I will refer to the concept of God in many ways such as: God, Source, Higher Self, Self, Higher Spiritual Self, Brahmin, God-Self, etc. They all mean the same thing: universal spirit.

why it's called the path to self-realization. But once you attain the self-realized state, your yoga practice becomes irrelevant. You no longer need to do yoga; you are yoga.

The Purpose of the Yoga Sutras

The Yoga Sutras help the seeker answer common questions such as, *Why am I here? What is my purpose? Why do humans suffer? And why do we die?*

Innately, you know that you are more than this human body. Whether religious or not, questions will arise throughout your lifetime, leading you to your soul's existence. On some level, you know you're a spiritual being having a human experience. But your daily life doesn't answer the ageless and timeless question of "Why?"

The Buddha, Gautama Siddhartha, was born in India around 563 BCE and sought to solve this puzzle. Born into wealth and royalty, the Indian child was predicted to become a king or a monk. To prevent his son from becoming the latter, Siddhartha's father sheltered him from the outside world and all suffering. But even in his wealthy life, having been given everything he could ever desire, young Siddhartha wanted more. He had a beautiful wife and infant son but was still dissatisfied. One day, Siddhartha convinced his father to let him spend a day in the village outside the palace walls. His father, remembering the prophecy at Siddhartha's birth, made sure that everyone who was poor and sick left the village for the day. His son was not to see suffering. Despite his father's careful planning, Siddhartha saw a man with deep lines on his ashen face and eyes sunken with fever on the way back to the palace. Shocked, young Siddhartha asked his charioteer, "Why does this man look like that?" His charioteer answered, "That man is sick." He then explained that all men become sick and eventually die. Shortly thereafter, Siddhartha left his family to learn to go beyond age, sickness, and death. He walked to the edge of the forest, where he found a teacher to study yoga and meditation. The Buddha, well-known to Buddhists and people of all religions, was a simple man. He was a man on a quest for the knowledge of transcendence. That is why the Buddha's story resonates with so many; we all have an innate desire to access this knowledge.

The Yoga Sutras provide you with the template for transcendence. If you study and follow them, they work. However, the ultimate goal is not to adhere to and follow every rule. With practice, the Yoga Sutras become an automatic part of your daily life.

The Journey Inward Away from Suffering

While the Eight Limbs of Yoga give us moral and ethical parameters for living, the main focus of the Sutras, as you will see in subsequent chapters, is an inward journey away from suffering. According to the Yoga Sutras, when we live with inconsistent personal discipline, moral boundaries, or the concept of Self, we create karma. This karmic debt generates more chaos and disruption in our thought patterns as we are pulled to react rather than act. Our lives become a constant stream of fires to be extinguished, so we can never move toward stillness and experience true joy. The first two limbs of yoga work like an iron to smooth out the wrinkles of your best clothes so you can look and feel nice. After that, the focus of the remaining limbs is to take you on an inward journey to find the stillness that has been there all along.

Each limb is a progressive build-up toward that point of stillness. However, the destination is not the end. If you adhere to the Eight Limbs' practice, you may reach samadhi or enlightenment. But as in any human experience, its attainment is only temporary. The practitioner must know this. To be in this world and attain enlightenment allows you to go back and experience life at another level. Life and its experiences will still remain; only your perception of them will change.

Human Suffering in Modern Times

In modern times, human suffering is exacerbated in all forms. We live with violence and threats from external forces, but we also live with many forms of internal suffering. Humans have always known suffering. We've always been faced with internal questions related to our mortality. We've had the internal struggles of fitting into a tribe or society and the moral questions of choosing the right path. However, the most significant suffering we know today is that of isolation.

As our lives become easier and more convenient, we become more isolated. If you live in a developed country, you might not know what it's like to go hungry for long periods or to be without shelter. It's more likely that you have a decently furnished home, a vehicle, a television, and food in the fridge. The risk of isolation is even greater if you can work remotely. Electronic devices now take our tolls, check out our groceries, and deliver food to a locker where we can pick it up without human interaction. We can live thousands of miles away from family members and still communicate through a video app or cell phone, but we no longer feel them through the sense of touch. Then, as we sit with friends, family, and work colleagues, we are on our devices with headphones and not interacting much. In 2023, the U.S. Surgeon General published a report stating that we are in an epidemic of loneliness and social isolation.[2] Suffering has been a part of humanity, but now it's headed to a new level.

The effects of modern life make it the worst kind of suffering. Never before in modern history have we seen such an uptick in lifestyle illnesses, addiction, and suicide. In the United States alone, over 150 million Americans suffer from at least one chronic lifestyle illness, and that rate is growing by 7% per year. According to the Centers for Disease Control and Prevention (CDC), deaths by opioid overdose (prescription or illicit opioids) between the years 2015 and 2016 grew by 21.5%. In 2016 alone, drug overdoses took the lives of 63,632 Americans. In addition, according to the National Institute on Alcohol Abuse and Alcoholism (NIAAA), 88,000 Americans die yearly from alcohol-related causes, making it the third preventable cause of death after tobacco use and other lifestyle illnesses. Suicide is the 10th leading cause of death in the U.S., with a jump of 24% between the years 1999 and 2014, with the most significant rate of increase from 2006 forward. Given these statistical facts, I would surmise that the suffering of the Western world is of the worst kind and needs transcendence and redemption.

Through all of our self-soothing with food, drugs, alcohol, and boxed entertainment, we are searching for a connection outside of ourselves that was once partially satisfied by community or time spent in nature. Even then, humans still had a lot to overcome. Yet our current suffering has added layers we now need to uncover.

The Yoga Sutras teach that the solution to extinguish all suffering is within. When we discover our universal connection to everyone and everything, we cease to feel alone and disconnected. In the end, "dis-ease" is nothing but disconnection, first from ourselves and then from others.

Is Suffering Really Futile?

Great philosophers and thinkers, including Patanjali, continually explored ways to overcome human suffering. The Buddha's life and work were experiments in transcending suffering. While the Eight Limbs of Yoga were presented as a means to transcend human suffering, I'm offering another perspective. What if human suffering isn't futile at all?

That is not to say I enjoy suffering. In truth, if I were invited to a party and had the choice of being guaranteed a splendid time or a horrible one, I'm confident I would pick splendid. Yet, my most significant learning experiences have come out of suffering. Triumph is often well-earned when mired in a fair amount of discomfort or suffering.

To experience true joy, you must know suffering, for everything in this human existence works through its dualistic nature. For example, without pain, we cannot appreciate pleasure. And, if there were no death, we would have a hard time appreciating life. And so it goes. (To explore duality more deeply, read my book *Heal Yourself: A Return to Wholeness: The Integration of Body, Mind, Soul, and Spirit*.)

To that end, I suggest that the ancient sages and seers might have been short-sighted. We aren't trying to end all suffering; we are moving toward a more peaceful and connected inner experience as we move through life. We are already miles ahead of the curve if we strive for a more meaningful and less chaotic life experience.

That being said, with consistent practice of the Eight Limbs of Yoga, you will obtain greater inner peace overall. The drama of life will no longer affect you as if you were a piece of driftwood being tossed about by a raging river. You will learn to take the good and bad with grace and gratitude. You will learn to appreciate the present moment fully but not get caught up in it.

As far as suffering is concerned, mastery of the Yoga Sutras gives you conscious choice-making. Before the experience of enlightenment, you believe you are a victim of your experiences. After enlightenment, you realize you are the orchestrator of those same experiences. The choice is in how you choose to live them.

The Subtle Effects of Yoga Asana and Why You Deserve More

We are what our deep, driving desire is. As our deep, driving desire is, so is our will. As our will is, so is our deed. As our deed is, so is our destiny.

—*Brihadaranyaka Upanishad 4.4-5*

Through yoga asana, you've been gaining the benefits of a broader yoga practice without direct intention. Now that you've tasted yoga's subtle effects, perhaps it's your invitation to explore them more consciously.

Suppose you've been invited to a fabulous party by a very wealthy friend. You drive up to the mansion, completely blown away by its grandeur. As the attendant takes your car, you sheepishly walk in the front door, certain you don't belong there. But as you enter, you are warmly greeted by your host, who invites you to explore her home. As you stand in the entry hall, you're transfixed by the elaborate decor and the impeccable architecture. You observe a gorgeous bouquet spilling over an ornate table and smell tantalizing food from another room. Even though you've been invited to explore the other rooms, you remain in the foyer, stunned that this one room is bigger than your entire home. You slowly make your way around it, staring at the impressive paintings, running your fingers across the antique furniture, and admiring the fancy guests entering the front door. You want to explore the other rooms but hesitate. You only need to walk a little further to see more. But amid all this luxury, your mind takes over; *You don't really deserve to be here. Who are you to be able to experience such extravagance? Just stay here before you break something or say the wrong thing and get kicked out.* Although you'd love to explore the mansion, you stand frozen with fear of the unknown and not being worthy. Your desires to learn and know more are real. Your soul is calling you to this experience.

In your journey of expansion, I'll be your guide, the mansion's owner. I'm not the one who possesses it, but the one who has openly displayed the wealth for you to explore. I invite you to freely observe, experience, taste, and touch the layers of ancient wisdom tied to your yoga asana practice. If you're hesitant, allow me to help you overcome your trepidation by unveiling your readiness.

A Commitment to Learn and Apply These Principles

Like the yoga asanas, the other limbs of yoga are best learned by experience. You can intellectualize the concepts, but they're only nice ideas on a page if you don't put them into daily practice. The truth in these principles lies in seeing them come to life.

Perhaps the greatest aspect of the Eight Limbs of Yoga is that it's rooted in self-study. You can opt for a teacher or guide, but it's not necessary. The guidelines are there for you to practice at your own pace and refer to when needed. No one is looking over your shoulder, telling you what you're doing wrong or how to practice them. When you're committed, the Yoga Sutras open you to a world of self-discovery.

Commit to learning and applying one of the principles weekly or every few weeks. Focus on that principle, pondering it deeply as you go about your daily activities. Recovery groups have a saying that goes, "Progress and not perfection." Know that there is no perfection. You will see your progress the more you practice, but perfection is an unattainable goal. And the search for it can be just as damaging as inaction.

One value that has been lost in modern society is the value of commitment. If you can't commit to your own life, who else will? And how can you commit to other things if you can't commit to you? Commitment doesn't mean you'll always get it right. It often means you'll get it wrong much of the time. Commitment means not giving up. And when you feel you've mastered a skill, move on to the next. Soon thereafter, the discipline of your practice will show up in other areas of your life. Before you know it, you'll find yourself more poised, organized, reliable, and happy.

As for the suffering? In the end, you'll say, "Suffering? Bring it on. I eat suffering for lunch." And that, my friend, is yoga. To quote Nisargadatta Maharaj, "In my world, nothing ever goes wrong."

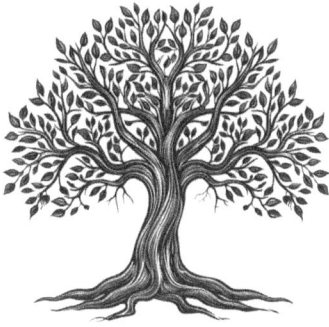

CHAPTER 1

The First Limb of Yoga

The Yamas

Some might say the world is going to hell in a handbasket. I would have to disagree. We are living in extraordinary times. Thousands of people have become more awakened in the past several years. They're beginning to question outdated and confining beliefs that were once deemed acceptable. They're pushing the limits to find new levels of acceptance for people of various beliefs and lifestyles.

On the other hand, we are living in a time of confusion, loneliness, and lack of fundamental moral precepts. With an increased number of people rejecting traditional religion and with the internet as a new god, many are inventing moral parameters as they go. When you take millions of people living in increased isolation and lacking direction through community sages or wisdom-filled elders, you get millions mindlessly paving the way forward. As a result, you come to a society of "everything goes," which ultimately doesn't work for the greater good.

Ethical and Moral Codes from the Past

Societies with strict rules and irrational or outdated laws are unfair to many. Religious organizations that exclude certain groups based on lifestyle or previous religious affiliation can seem mean and cruel. That being said, when we let the pendulum swing too far in the other direction, as we have in today's society, we get chaos, isolation, and a lack of moral direction.

Take the example of a toddler who has just learned to walk. That toddler needs his new-found freedom, but he also needs boundaries. He can't wander into a crowd, leaving his parents far behind. Even though he can now reach things higher up, attaining every object he reaches for can be catastrophic if he pulls on something heavy or sharp. Given his new abilities, he needs his caregivers to set limits until he can make safe choices.

Similarly, when we look back to the 1950s in the United States, for example, we see a different society than we have today. Many would agree it was too constricting and unfair and showed a lack of tolerance for major groups such as women and African Americans. That is true. Yet, delving into a recently past society can also show us what good came from it. After World War II ended, U.S. citizens had a sense of solidarity.

The main focus was creating solid families, neighborhoods, and communities. Although many women worked out of necessity during wartime, they stayed at home to raise children post-war. As a result, women had extensive networks of other women to rely on for support. In general, neighborhoods were places where children felt safe growing up. They could roam the neighborhoods on bikes or play outside until dark. Bigger families meant more chores and more responsibilities. Therefore, kids learned the value of hard work. Jobs were more secure. And most understood that a strong work ethic would solidify your future. Free time was spent at church picnics, walks in the park, or afternoons at the library. Families pooled together to help each other and pitched in when a neighbor was sick or had a new baby. While the 1950s American society was not ideal in every sense, most lived within the boundaries of a personal and societal moral code.

The Search for Moral and Ethical Parameters

Today's multicultural society will never look like the U.S. of the 1950s, nor would many agree it should. While we don't all share the same religious, moral, or ethical parameters, we share the need for something more profound. I look around at many people today, especially Millennials and Zoomers, and see that they crave connection and community. I also see the need for direction and boundaries that make sense for them in their modern world. Without direction, we can't expect to see great leaders in the future. The confining boundaries of tribal life, for example, make tribe members blindly follow their tribe leader. But at least there is leadership and, oftentimes, the wisdom to lead. Yet, suppose we were to take the millions of youth today with no leadership or moral direction and let them fend for themselves. What would arise instead would be selfish and narcissistic people who have difficulty leading. Unfortunately, we have seen this happen already.

The invention and advancement of the internet have been both a source of liberation and serious moral and ethical problems. Many children today learn to surf the net before they can run or have developed speech. Yet they're faced with images and dialogue that put ethical matters into question before proper brain development allows them to choose between right and wrong. While I'm a big YouTube fan and a YouTuber, many children are drawn to prominent YouTubers who use profane language as part of their online persona. Even though my son was twelve when he started watching YouTube and was already hearing profanity in middle school, I know many younger kids who watch the same videos. And that is but one example. Smartphones have allowed teens to be connected via text, email, and social media. But it has also opened them up to cyberbullying and imprudent sexual behavior, such as sexting, that they deem as harmless but that can have incriminating consequences.

Modern living doesn't only affect the budding morality of children and teens but also adults. For example, on the subject of fidelity in marriage and committed monogamous relationships, what was once well-understood is now confusing and fuzzy. Couples are now faced with deciding whether a social media connection with a previous lover is cheating or if frequent texting with a "good friend" can be conceived as going outside of the relationship. Then there are the questions of whether or not illegal downloading of media content is stealing, and the list goes on.

While loose ethical and moral boundaries are certainly not the fault of Millennials, Zoomers, or any specific generation, they result from modern social conditions such as the high divorce rate, the breakdown in local communities, and increasing social isolation due to people living life through a computer screen. In many ways, morality has become a free-for-all. At the same time, people crave moral and ethical parameters in some form. On the other hand, whose guidance can you trust if you're searching for moral and ethical guidance?

I once read that the fastest growing group of Atheists are Zoomers or those under the age of twenty-eight, as of 2025. While I agree that religions don't have all the answers, having no ethical and moral direction or code for living isn't the answer either. Whether you grew up Christian, Jewish, Muslim, Buddhist, Hindu, or in any other faith or without faith, today's modern living can shake up your moral and ethical parameters like no other modern time. We live in a time of relativity. Moral and ethical boundaries seem to move in every situation and circumstance.

The Eight Limbs of Yoga's guidelines have been time-tested for close to two thousand years. Like many philosophical principles on ethical and moral living, the Yamas and Niyamas overlap with guidelines from many religions and philosophies. Many have a distaste for religion or find inconsistencies with the manufactured rules drawn from religious texts. These principles outlined by Patanjali aren't religious yet have the power to pull the student to their inner power to make decisions based on truth. At that point, the student ceases to rely on others' input or dogma to decide how to act or who to be but will draw from their inner wisdom. Through disciplined practice, the need for parameters falls away as the student becomes the wisdom.

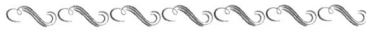

The 1st Yama

Ahimsa: Non-Harming

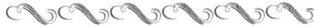

When negative thoughts arise or when one feels compelled to commit acts of violence out of greed, anger, or delusion and indulged with mild, moderate, or extreme intensity—-they are based on ignorance and are sure to cause pain. At such times, think of their opposites.—Yoga Sutra 2-34

In the presence of one firmly established in nonviolence, all hostilities cease. - Yoga Sutra 2-35

As put forth by Patanjali, the goal of ahimsa is as follows: *When the vow of ahimsa is established in someone, all enmity ceases in his or her presence because that per-*

son emits harmonious vibrations.[3] This means that when non-harming or non-violence is practiced continuously in thought, word, and deed, you begin to vibrate on a level where violence can't exist around you.

In our modern world, violence seems to be everywhere. However, we have become accustomed to and perhaps numb to the violent acts that occur daily. Violence is perpetuated in all forms of media, making companies wealthy through clicks, views, and advertising dollars. When you see or hear stories of violence, you may voice your disgust and search for answers. In a knee-jerk reaction, you run through the list: Must I blame society, guns, violent video games, the breakdown of family and community, or the politicians? Depending on the strength of your reaction, you may even collaborate with like-minded individuals and generate discussions, protests, and marches to stop that form of violence. You may even consider yourself a non-violent person and insist: *It's the other guy, not me or anyone I know.*

The yogic way views violence differently. The Yoga Sutras consider that anyone who has one thought of harm generated toward another, either dormant or active, has violence within them.

Here are a couple of examples:

Have you or anyone you know ever taken pleasure in watching reality television?

Reality shows are filled with violence, though you might not have considered them in that way. Even romantic reality shows highlight a "villain" and are edited to display the most turbulent couples who fight, scream, and create discord for the other players.

Do you enjoy rooting for your favorite sports team?

You create animosity toward the opposing team when you get into competitive fandom. You find fault with certain players and want them to lose or get injured so your team has a fighting chance. Some sports fans get so revved up during games they initiate fights, taking it personally if their team loses.

Here are some examples that will undoubtedly hit home.

- Do you ever get upset when some idiot driver cuts you off?
- Are you irritated when the checkout person takes longer than expected?
- Do your spouse, children, boss, or neighbors get on your nerves?
- Do you ever have negative self-talk?

If you answered "yes" to any or all of the above, congratulations! You are human.

From the illustrated examples, can you see how living a life of non-harming or non-violence can be tricky?

And yet, most often, we've been looking at violence from the wrong angle.

Violence or thoughts of violence begin with you. I understand the harshness of this statement. But keep an open mind as we explore the yogic path on this subject.

In writing this, I'm reminded of a song I sang as a child in my church choir. The title is "Let There Be Peace on Earth," written by Jill Jackson-Miller and Sy Miller. The song begins with this stanza, "Let there be peace on earth, and let it begin with me. Let there be peace on earth. The peace that was meant to be." The song emphasizes that peace, in other words, non-violence, must begin with you and me. The second stanza continues, "With God as our father. Brothers, all are we. Let me walk with my brother in perfect harmony." We are all brothers and sisters as one humanity. So, who does that leave out?

To illustrate this further, an ancient Objiwa Indian saying states, "No tree has branches so foolish as to fight among themselves." We are all together as parts of the same tree, interconnected by deep roots. Yet, we have lost sight of this interconnectedness.

Here is a real-life example from nature. Pando is the world's largest aspen tree in Utah. On the surface, it appears to be 47,000 trees with trunks, branches, and leaves. But Pando is one tree connected by a singular root system. Pando means interconnected. If we look at the symbolism, we can remember our deep connection to one another. This makes the principle of ahimsa easier to comprehend.

When you have a violent thought toward anyone or anything, including yourself, you have the potential to harm. In the yoga sutras 2-33 and 2-34, Patanjali suggests choosing an opposite thought to the negative one to turn it around. What Patanjali means is that we don't want to feed harmful thoughts, which can lead to harmful actions. We want to starve the negative thought when it's barely forming.

In truth, negative thoughts are natural. Your human brain is hard-wired for survival and looks for danger whenever it can. Living through the principle of ahimsa means bringing awareness to your thoughts, words, intentions, behaviors, or actions that can harm you or another.

Fear as the Driving Force to Violence

All violence comes from fear. Those who study the Eight Limbs of Yoga learn to turn fear into unconditional love. Unconditional love comes from a place of compassion and oneness. Oftentimes, you don't know the whole story behind why someone does something; therefore, it's best not to judge.

I recently attended an Abraham-Hicks workshop. During the seminar, Abraham said, "Give others the benefit of the doubt." This simple statement spoke volumes. I interpreted it to mean that instead of thinking negatively about others, I should consider that I don't know their whole story. A couple of decades ago, I learned a similar tactic called Making up the Story.

Making up the story means creating other realities for a person when you aren't aware of their reality. So, for the person who cuts you off while driving, you might think:

Well, maybe their wife is in labor and must get to a hospital.

Or perhaps they really need to go to the restroom.

Or maybe their boss is screaming at them to get back to work.

When you create a story about someone with several possibilities, you give them the benefit of the doubt. This fosters more compassion. By doing this, you don't get angry or upset. In fact, the opposite happens; you want them to go ahead of you. It's a great game to play.

Self-Discovery Through Ahimsa

Ahimsa starts within. It begins with our self-talk, sense of self-worth, and how we treat ourselves. I hear many people who berate and put themselves down. That is violence toward oneself. Treating yourself with kindness is ahimsa. Give yourself a break when you've done something wrong or said the wrong thing. Stop berating yourself. Get the lesson and move on. Talk to yourself like you would a close friend.

In *The Four Agreements*, Don Miguel Ruiz writes, "Humans punish themselves endlessly for not being what they believe they should be. They become very self-abusive and use other people to abuse themselves as well. But nobody abuses us more than we abuse ourselves." Treating yourself with kindness can help you be more compassionate with others.

Often, mothers sacrifice themselves for their children. They dress their children in beautiful clothing while they deny themselves. Or they feel bad for wanting a night out with friends. Allow yourself to receive what you want, need, and desire. You will have more to give your children and others once you do.

Fulfilling your own needs helps you honor ahimsa. Often, aggressive or violent words are a result of self-denial. When you deny your needs, they become suppressed. And when they become suppressed, anger ensues. Needs must be fulfilled; when they aren't, they become loud like a hungry child. Take care of yourself first. Get the proper amount of sleep, food, water, and exercise. As a yogi practicing ahimsa, try to abstain from harmful substances such as tobacco, alcohol, and drugs. Surround yourself with supportive friends, loved ones, and peers. Make sure you get twelve hugs a day, as Dr. Leo Buscaglia used to say, even if it's from your cat.

Notice Your Mind and Thoughts

The next step in attaining the benefits of ahimsa is to analyze your mind and thoughts. Patanjali said, "When you are steadfast in your abstention of thoughts of harm directed toward yourself and others, all living creatures will cease to feel fear in your presence." That means all of your consistent thoughts must be nonviolent. Understandably, this is not an easy feat.

Our minds tend to be cluttered with thoughts, many of which are violent. It may be subtle, such as muttering to yourself, *I will kill him if he says that again.* Even if the intent is never to kill, the thought moves toward inflicting harm or ill will on another. Thoughts such as, "I'll never get rid of this illness," Or, "I'll always be fat," can also be considered harmful. Defeatist thoughts cause you to believe that your body should remain unwell.

When I observed my thoughts, I noticed I have a terrible habit of thinking negatively about other drivers. If someone cuts me off the highway or won't let me in a lane, I mindlessly shout out, "Stupid person!" When I first noticed this, I was shocked. It had become an unconscious habit, and the reaction was automatic. Since then, I've tried to be mindful and not react that way.

Notice Your Words

Since thoughts and speech are so intricately intertwined, the practice of ahimsa is carried out in our words. I'm not sure why the expression, "Sticks and stones may break my bones, but names will never hurt me," ever came about. Nothing could be further from the truth. Injury through words is the kind that cuts the deepest, and memories of verbal injury tend to remain. Most of us have little awareness of what we say and are oblivious to whether our words might harm others. Often, we brush it off by saying, "Oh, I was just being helpful." Or "I was only kidding."

Children and adolescents can be cruel to each other, but adults can be cruel too. As adults, we teach our children to speak kindly to one another by reprimanding or insisting. But children learn more from our actions than from verbal warnings. They also hear your intent through non-verbal cues. Children are perceptive, and they can tell if you walk your talk.

Unfortunately, we're usually more comfortable saying hurtful things to family and friends. The subconscious safety net with a loved one somehow permits us to say more, even if it's misguided or unkind. We must learn to extend kindness to our family and friends even if our comfort level has lowered barriers and made us more vulnerable. The same rules of compassion and unconditional love must extend to all beings, whether they're close to you or not.

You may have said something hurtful to someone, and for you, it has been long forgotten. But that wound might still be open for the receiver of the insult or harmful words. It's easy to say, "Oh, don't be so sensitive." But the principle of ahimsa holds us responsible for the intent to injure or harm.

While studying at the Chopra Center, my teacher, Dr. David Simon, taught a beautiful way to observe your words before speaking them. It's called the Three Gateways to Speech. Before speaking, ask yourself three things. *Is what I'm about to say true?* If the answer is yes, move on to the next gateway. The second gateway is, *Is what I'm about to say necessary?* If the answer is yes, move on to the third gateway, *Is what I'm about to say, kind?* If you pass through all three gateways, you know you're speaking from a place of non-harming.

Another form of harmful speech is gossip. You can cause harm when you talk negatively about others, even if you don't know them.

When I'm mindful, I have observed that gossip is a problem for me. I'm a writer, author, and storyteller. It can be easy for me to tell stories about people who aren't present. With my gift of gab, I'm trying to be more mindful of spinning a story in a more positive light, giving a person the benefit of the doubt instead of seeking the entertainment value. One way I can do this is to ask permission. Even if it doesn't put them in the best light, I'm not creating more harm in telling their story.

Notice Your Actions

The principle of ahimsa asks us not to create or support any physical acts of violence and, in the purest sense, not killing animals for meat. Modifications of this principle for Western living may be made, and our conscious awareness can be shifted to remain sensitive to the animal that has given up its life for food. For example, in keeping with the principle of ahimsa, you can minimize your meat consumption to once a week. You can also choose meat from sources that have been kind to the animals. Look for organic and animal welfare ratings on your meat and dairy products. Choose organic fruit, vegetables, and grains as much as possible. Additionally, you can refrain from using harmful chemicals in your home to clean and eliminate pests.

Remember the Golden Rule: *Treat others as you would like to be treated*, and extend this treatment to your family, friends, strangers, animals, and the environment.

☙ Living Ahimsa off the Mat ❧

To live ahimsa off the mat, commit to these statements for a day at a time.

1. I will listen to my inner dialogue. I will notice harmful thoughts toward myself or others.
2. I will meet my needs by eating healthfully, staying hydrated, getting fresh air, and exercising.
3. I will declare today a violence-free media day. I will abstain from watching the news, reading about violent acts, watching violent shows, or playing violent games.
4. I will observe my words and stop myself when I think they may cause injury or harm.
5. I will refrain from gossip.
6. I will use my arms and hands to spread love instead of hate. Today, I will give hugs, write a love letter, send a thank you note, or plant a flower or garden. I will sow the seeds of love, knowing that nonviolence starts with me.

☙ Practicing Ahimsa on the Mat ❧

In your yoga asana practice, treat yourself with loving kindness. Many people practice hot or intense yoga and feel they must "tough it out." Toughing it out is not ahimsa. Listen to your body during every pose. Look for signs of over-stress in your muscles and joints while getting into and holding the pose. Stop if a pose is hurting or if you feel a sharp pain. Practicing ahimsa means lying in *savasana*, relaxation pose, if you feel too tired or stressed in a yoga class. Give yourself permission to honor your body's inner wisdom.

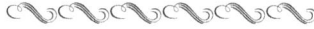

~~~~~~~~~~

The 2nd Yama

Satya: Truthfulness

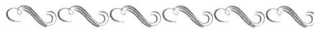

~~~~~~~~~~

Truth is victorious, never untruth. Truth is the way; truth is the goal of life. Reached by sages who are free from self-will. —The Mundaka Upanishad, Part III—1.5

To one firmly established in truthfulness, his word becomes binding on objective reality. —Yoga Sutra 2-36

This Yoga Sutra makes some incredible promises. It states that when yogis are established in *satya*, truthfulness, they obtain instant manifestation power. In other words, they receive the benefits of hard work without the work. Let's analyze the deeper meaning of this sutra.

The ultimate goal of yoga is to realize your true nature: oneness with God, and that you are Source Energy or the Self (as repeated throughout The Upanishads, meaning higher spiritual self) in physical form. Furthermore, your self-realization must come from the experience of absolute absorption with the Self. According to The Upanishads, that is the only truth that exists. If you have experiential knowledge of oneness and can access it at will, you have obtained all there is to know.

In the introduction to the Mundaka Upanishad, author Eknath Easwaran writes, *Satyam eva jayate nanritam*— "Truth alone prevails, not unreality." Unreality is anything that changes. Reality is that which never changes.

Therefore, if you stand in the truth of who you are at all times, you are vibrating at God-consciousness. As you vibrate in God-consciousness, you can create or manifest anything you desire.

In *Demystifying Patanjali*, Swami Kriyananda says that all words have power when you attune your awareness to the highest octave of what is. In doing that, your verbal expressions come through the blissful state of God-consciousness.

Practical Satya

Remaining truthful to oneself and others is a tough challenge. Try going an entire day without lying, deceiving, or stretching the truth. It's an eye-opening experiment. I thought I was extremely honest until I observed every word and thought for a day. I discovered that, for various reasons, I diverged from truthful speech and thought on several occasions.

Patajali suggests that we speak truth except for harming another person, leading us back to the principle of ahimsa. He encourages silence instead of speaking untruth or a truth that injures or harms.

Does Dishonesty Make You Bad or Evil?

Since humans are prone to deception and lies, are we inherently bad or immoral? Our propensity to stretch the truth, tell "white" lies, or lie outright is often to conceal a painful truth we would prefer to keep inside. A child learns quickly how to lie to protect himself from the painful consequences of punishment. Lies can undoubtedly be the product of an immoral person. However, most of us deceive out of fear of not being good enough, of what others might think, of negative consequences, or others' reactions.

When I first tried online dating a few years back, I created an authentic profile. However, I discovered that many men had no problem creating deceitful profiles. Their dishonesty disturbed me because the truth usually emerges once you meet them. So why did these people lie? Were they bad people? Some might be innately dishonest, but most probably feared not being good enough.

Another reason people deceive is to keep the peace. This is dangerous because lying to keep the peace often leads to further deception.

Parents also teach children to deceive by not accepting the truth of who they are. Some parents would rather have their children fit into a mold than allow them to express themselves authentically. For a parent, sometimes the truth is hard to accept. If you have your heart set on your little boy becoming a star athlete and he prefers to paint, you may be disappointed. As a parent of three, there were many truths I didn't want to face. However, not facing them created a rift in the relationship. Quiet deception is often more damaging than a booming truth.

Using Authenticity to Gauge the Truth

Many believe that white lies are not deceitful and don't hurt anyone. But truthfulness is more about creating authenticity in relationships and with yourself.

Authentic self-expression strengthens bonds with the people around you and helps you live a more expansive life.

For example, in Ayurvedic consultations, I used to talk to clients about their health habits. Many tended to sugarcoat their health and lifestyle choices until I asked deeper questions. On the surface, clients would claim they were very healthy. However, upon digging deeper, I found they didn't sleep well, exercised little, or had a poor diet. Often, the refusal to be honest with themselves caused one or more of their health problems.

When you're deceitful, you'll know even if the person doesn't find out. You will carry that burden, weighing you down more than what you lied about. Remember, yoga is about uniting every part of you. When untruths are present, you divide instead of unite.

Accepting others' truths can help us expand unity consciousness. Perhaps you've gotten angry when a friend or a loved one revealed a truth you didn't want to hear. You may have needed to know, but you didn't handle it well. Handling your disappointments and negative feelings can open the door to authenticity.

Fears of Telling the Truth

We can perpetuate deceit through our fears. For example, if your child tells you about something they've done and you react poorly, you unknowingly ask them to lie next time. Fearful of your reaction, the child will go into self-preservation mode and not tell the truth. Parents sometimes overreact or react without love. Practicing satya might help you revisit the conversation and let them know that telling the truth is safe.

The fear of someone's reaction also tends to happen among couples. For example, the wife spends too much money at the mall and is afraid to tell her husband until the credit card bill arrives. Or the husband wants to spend time with the guys after work but fears his wife's reaction, so he tells her he's working late. In an ideal world, love would transcend fear, and everyone could take ownership of their truth.

Be gracious to others who speak the truth. It can be difficult to reveal your innermost thoughts, experiences, or past actions. When a friend or loved one is brave enough to share, that information must be met with the least amount of judgment to keep satya flowing. And then, when it's your turn to share, your loved one may be more open to receiving it without judgment.

❧ Living Satya off the Mat ❧

To live satya off the mat, implement the following statements for a day or a week.

1. I will watch my thoughts and notice when I tend toward dishonesty or when I'm about to tell an untruth. I will also observe why I'm choosing deception over truth.
2. I will notice my reaction to others when they speak the truth. Am I unloving, harsh, or judgmental in response? If I choose to remain silent, does my facial expression or body language tell the person I don't accept their truth?
3. I will make sure that the truth I speak will not harm others. I know it's better to stay silent than to cause harm through my words.
4. I will mentally review the last seven days and note any untruthfulness or inauthenticity. I will then make amends and correct my mistakes to live satya more fully.

❧ Practicing Satya on the Mat ❧

Listen to your body during your yoga asana practice. Be truthful with yourself about your limitations. Don't push yourself into a pose or variation of it if you're not ready.

You might be tired today and need to take it easy. Or perhaps you've been inactive for several days, and now is the time to challenge yourself. Being honest with yourself doesn't mean to give in to your current state. If you're feeling sad, depressed, or stressed, it's reasonable to want to feel better. Honesty means greeting your body and mind where they are today. When you're grounded in the truthfulness of your state, you can set the intention for a better one.

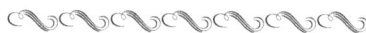

⌇⌇⌇⌇⌇⌇⌇⌇⌇

The 3rd Yama

Asteya: Non-Stealing

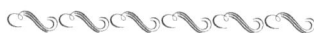

⌇⌇⌇⌇⌇⌇⌇

To one established in non-stealing, all wealth comes. - Yoga Sutra 2.37

Many have heard the commandment, "Thou shalt not steal," from the Bible. Yet, in modern times, the concept of stealing has become fuzzy. Before apps like Spotify, Pandora, and Apple Music, you could download music, movies, software, and video games for free on torrent websites. Many people in my family felt fine downloading these items. I felt uneasy and often spoke loudly about it. To me, downloading material you would typically have to pay for is stealing. Now, most people freely use the internet to post and download all kinds of content with no qualms. The argument I often hear is, "Everyone does it." Or, "These people are charging too much, so I feel it is my right to download it for free." This only perpetuates poverty consciousness.

To Steal or Not to Steal?

My personal opinions aside, let's explore why people might be inclined to take what doesn't belong to them.

Some people steal for entertainment value, but those are the minority. Others steal out of necessity. For example, a mother living in the streets might steal food to feed her children. Some might say this is rightful stealing. But most people steal because of jealousy, envy, or greed.

Jealousy, Envy, and Greed

While jealousy, envy, and greed are common emotional states, they are all rooted in lack. For example, if you're jealous of someone's wealth, fame, or marital status, you might believe you can't have what that person has. That is a lack mentality. Envy resonates similarly. If you see someone with a Maserati, and it's a car you've had your eye on, you might be envious that they have it and you don't. And if you feel you must steal from the rich to give to the poor, you're operating in the mentality of greed. While the intention might seem righteous, the belief is that the rich person doesn't deserve to be rich and that it's your job to establish equilibrium. And that is greed and pride.

Most people wouldn't go to great lengths to steal from others, but what about subtle ways? A person who sleeps with a married person, not in an open marriage, is stealing a marital partner. If you run with a business idea that your friend first had, you are stealing his idea. And if you fill your purse with six miniature bottles of jam at brunch, you're stealing. In other words, you're communicating to the universe, "I don't trust you'll give me what I need."

Wealth Is Your Birthright

You came into this abundant world as Source energy in physical form. The world has everything you need for your physical journey. There is no lack. When you're disconnected from God and the world, it feels like you're in the middle of the ocean, drowning, with no lifeboat. This disconnection causes you to take hold of anything you can to survive. But if you remain in this mindset, you will never thrive.

Have you ever noticed that the rich do, in fact, get richer, and the poor get poorer? It's not for the reasons you think. The rich aren't somehow sucking up all the riches. The poor tend to remain in a poverty mindset with feelings of lack, jealousy, envy, and greed, and the rich, while some might be greedy, have figured out how to overcome the feelings of lack.

You'll understand what I mean if you drive through a poor town or inner city. You will notice graffiti, property damage, clutter, and filth everywhere. Those things are not the result of rich people going to those neighborhoods, destroying property, and leaving trash; it's the result of the angry, jealous, envious, and greedy who choose to act out in a manner that perpetuates the poorness they are trying to get away from.

I was talking with a high-functioning autistic woman who was excited about getting a rent-controlled apartment in Orange County, California. She was ecstatic about getting this apartment but commented that her rent-controlled building had tons of theft. Another person I spoke to, who lives in a rent-controlled apartment in San Francisco, told a similar story. She revealed that the residents use the back of the building as a city dump. They have been given the opportunity to pay a fraction of the rent costs in these areas and yet have no appreciation for what they have. Instead, they choose to steal from their neighbors and trash their residences.

Not Taking More Than You Need

You can expand asteya to mean not taking more than you need. For example, you might feel you can take as much as you want at a buffet, even though you can't finish it all. In your poverty mindset, you think, *After all, I paid for it, so I should get my fair share.* Another example might be taking a large stack of napkins at a restaurant when you only need one or two. Or, suppose you're at a hotel with complimentary breakfast, and you can't resist stuffing your bag with goodies for the rest of your day.

I remember the early 1980s when Cabbage Patch dolls were a hot item. Around Christmas time, when a new shipment arrived, the dolls would fly off the shelves. Because of people's greed, many children who wanted the doll couldn't get it. It's a silly example, indeed. However, you can apply this self-centered act to other occasions as well. Have you ever tried to buy a snow shovel after a big blizzard or toilet paper in 2020? You might argue that these actions aren't stealing. We live in a capitalistic society, and buying things in excess is your right. Or is it? Just because you can doesn't mean you should. When someone purchases all the front-row seats to a concert and then sells them at an astronomical price to make a significant profit, is it right? Asteya teaches that it's not. When you're filled with greed and take something because it's there, that is stealing.

An Abundance Mindset

In the Yoga Sutra 2.37, Patanjali makes a grand claim: *If you stop taking, wealth will come to you.* In other words, if you chase wealth, it evades you. But if you stop chasing it, it will chase you.

It all comes down to mindset. If you are the poorest person on the planet but believe you have everything, all wealth is yours. And if you have some money but believe others are constantly taking your opportunities for more wealth, you will always remain poor.

In your abundance mindset, you trust that the world will always provide for you. Your focus is no longer on lack but on the wealth that surrounds you. When I began to shift toward wealth consciousness in 2013, I was listening to Tony Robbins' audio program, *Get the Edge*. He demonstrated how wealthy we already are with public libraries containing all the world's knowledge for free. Nature's abundance is all around us. Look at the plants, trees, animals, and fertile soil. They are constantly abundantly growing. One year, I planted a tiny mint plant, and without any care, it overtook my garden. Additionally, most of us don't have to hunt and kill for food anymore; we just go to the grocery store.

Modern plumbing is an invention I appreciate. I feel abundantly wealthy that I can sit on a toilet and flush it without worrying about where the waste is headed. I also enjoy a hot shower daily. If I were born in 1850 instead of 1970, I wouldn't have the luxury of my life-style today.

We take for granted many things that make life abundant in modern times. Learning to appreciate abundance in things unrelated to dollars in your bank account can help you move closer to releasing a lack mentality.

Many people think thoughts of poverty out of hab-it. This habit is so hard-wired that they hardly notice when complaining about what they don't have instead of appreciating what they do have. For example, one of my friends spent eighteen months searching for a job. During that time, he was depressed and desperate, stating that if only he could get a job, any job, he'd be grateful. Now he has two jobs, and he still complains. He complains he has no time and that things cost too much. Some people never learn to appreciate, so they remain poor whether they have money or not.

Joyful gratitude is the key to abundance. You won't feel envy, jealousy, or greed when you remain joyfully grateful for everything you have. Furthermore, you will be happy for others when they receive wealth, happiness, and abundance.

❦ Living Asteya off the Mat ❧

In everyday situations, practice taking only what you need. That doesn't mean you can't drive an expensive car or have lavish goals for your future. It means holding onto the mindset that there is always enough to go around. Practice abundance consciousness daily in mundane events such as waiting in line. If someone tries to take over your lane while driving, let them. Or if someone tries to take your parking space, allow them to take it. Another one will open up because abundance is everywhere. When you let go of the notion "I must get mine before someone else does," all wealth comes to you. Living like this, in all ways, will allow you to feel abundant and whole because you hold the secret to abundance.

❦ Practicing Asetya on the Mat ❧

In yoga class, some people can get possessive about their specific spot in class or the space around them. If you enter the class and someone is already in your spot, try to hold onto an abundance mindset. If the class is crowded, repeat silently. There is enough space for everyone. Move your mat or turn to the side during class so the students next to you can get into the pose. Instead of saving spots for your friends, allow others to fill in. Remember that yoga is an individual practice. You can always see your friends after class.

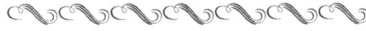

CRITERIA

The 4th Yama

Brahmacharya: Self-Control

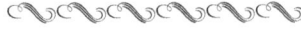

It is the mind that frees us or enslaves. Driven by the senses, we become bound; Master of the senses, we become free. Those who seek freedom must master the senses. -Amrita-bindu Upanishad, verses 2 & 3

One who is established in continence (sexual restraint) gains vitality.—Yoga Sutra 2:38

The fourth yama can be confusing for the modern yogi. After reading several translations and interpretations of *brahmacharya*, I'd like to offer different practical and spiritual perspectives.

When Patanjali composed the Yoga Sutras, it was common practice for men to go into the forests of India to study with a teacher and learn the ways of spiritual life. Most often, these young men wouldn't remain in the forest with their gurus forever. They would spend twelve years studying the Vedas and learning the ways of yogic life, and then they would return home to get married. As students, they practiced celibacy. It was thought that semen retention led to greater mental clarity. However, living a chaste life was never meant to be repression. Brahmacharya was taught to help spiritual students learn the value of sense control and apply it when returning home.

Since sexual desire is one of the most potent energies we possess, it's interesting to explore the value of harnessing its power toward a higher good. And gaining control over our senses can help us mindfully choose proper thought and action.

Expression and Not Suppression

I would like to open this exploration by pointing out the following: *That which is suppressed becomes distorted.* For hundreds of years (if not thousands), the subject of sex has been a taboo. In modern times, anything surrounding the subject of sex can conjure up feelings of shame, guilt, embarrassment, and avoidance. Many religions have taught that sex is evil, immoral, or sinful outside of marriage. Furthermore, in the studies of the Yoga Sutras, some authors have interpreted sex as being purely functional for the purpose of procreation, with all other desires being bad as they keep us in bondage. These interpretations remind me of strict Biblical teachings. But we can also attribute it to many religions that regard sex as shameful.

Yet, we have seen what suppression of sexual desires does when it rears its ugly head. Every day, we hear stories about people taking advantage of others sexually. The shame surrounding sexual desires allows deviant behavior to perpetuate.

In the past couple of years, I've had discussions with a couple of men in their twenties who heard about celibacy and semen retention through social media influencers. I saw one of them a year after he decided to try this experiment. As it turns out, toward the end of that year, he was having an affair with a married woman and obsessively having sex with her. Another man I spoke to, who was celibate for religious reasons, kept company with a woman from his church. But after being friends for some time, they caved into having sex with each other and felt enormous shame and guilt afterward. This man told me that no matter how much they tried to follow celibacy (so they wouldn't go to hell), they kept "accidentally" having sex with each other.

As you may have guessed, the suppression of desire never works.

While the Vedas might view desire as undesired, the Buddha discovered through trial and error that one can never eliminate it.

Built into our human perspective is the need to have desires. The desire to breathe, eat, drink water, sleep, and eliminate is essential to life. But so is sexual desire. If humans were designed to procreate only during mating season, as some species do, we would have no desire for sex outside of mating. And yet, that isn't the case. So, our sexual desire is good and whole, as is the desire to eat, drink, and sleep.

But where it gets complicated is when we let our desires run rampant like a starving fox in a forest.

Because of suppressed sexual desire, many people react with retaliatory thoughts and behaviors. For example, as a teenage girl, you might have screamed at your mom, "You can't tell me what to wear! I'll wear this mini-skirt and low-cut blouse if I want to!" Or if you were a teenage boy with a budding sexual curiosity but couldn't easily talk about it with your parents or siblings, you may have gotten addicted to porn. Perhaps you were raised religiously and taught that you couldn't have sex before marriage. So when you got to college, you slept with as many people as you could.

In today's dating world, promiscuity is almost expected before meeting face-to-face. Recently, I joined a dating app. After texting with a guy a few times, he asked, "How do you feel about spicy pics?" While I was put off, I wasn't shocked. Many men on dating apps expect that women will send revealing photos because they do.

On a practical level, brahmacharya, as the interpretation of self-control or sexual restraint, would be the modern-day phrase "Keep it in your pants!" All joking aside, that is the intent. Just because we have the desire doesn't mean we need to act on it. And just because we have the thought doesn't mean we need to keep entertaining that thought. We have a choice.

If we consider a desire as neutral, not good or bad, we remove the shame from it. In that way, it won't be distorted.

So what is the solution? Distract yourself or change your focus.

Suppose you're on a road trip and get the urge to use the restroom. Then, to your dismay, you discover that the next exit is twenty miles away. Knowing how far it is only makes matters worse. All you can think about is peeing. As you sit groaning with your legs crossed, a fellow passenger comes to the rescue and distracts you by putting on music or playing a car game. By the time you finally get to the exit, you forget you have to go.

That's how you shift focus. You do it all of the time.

You give into certain desires and refrain from others. That is how you master proper discernment. No matter what modern society dictates, you don't need to have sex after the fourth date or send naked pictures to a person you barely know. You don't have to look at porn or be considered a prude, or make sexual jokes at another's expense. You could, however. But as a Brahmacharyi or one who practices brahmacharya, you are learning to hold back when appropriate.

Flowing with God

That leads to the spiritual interpretation of brahmacharya: *to flow with Brahma* (God or the Creative Force). I hadn't learned this translation in my yoga teacher training, but I feel it has better resonance than restraint, the most commonly used translation.

Ponder that for a moment, "To flow with God." When you flow with God, life is easy. You're not fighting against your desires or caving in with fear, shame, and guilt. As you flow with God, you will always know which action or thought is appropriate.

Sexual energy in its purest form is creative. The creative essence that flows through you is God-force energy. Therefore, why would you try to suppress or feel ashamed of a God-given gift?

Women who have carried a baby and given birth know this first hand. Their body is a wellspring of creation as they feel the growing baby inside. It's awe-inspiring to witness the formation of life through the sexual impulse.

Creative or Source energy is available to all of us. We are creative beings who are meant to create. As author Eknath Easwaran wrote in his translation and commentary on The Upanishads, "Sexual desire, like everything else in The Upanishads, is only partly physical. Essentially, it is a spiritual force—pure, high-octane energy— and brahmacharya means its transformation."

Holding Back for Perfect Timing

Let's suppose you're building a house. To that end, you hire an architect, contractors, and an interior designer. Building a house takes a lot of planning and preparation before you can break ground. The architect must finish the plans, the contractors must get the proper permits and building materials, and the weather conditions must be favorable to start with the foundation. But what if you rush the process in your haste to get your home done? For example, you might accept a sloppy architectural plan, ask the contractors to skip the permits, and give them an unrealistic deadline to break ground. If you were to rush the creative process, you would generate problems that may not have occurred had you been patient and honored the logical steps forward.

The practice of brahmacharya can help you avoid unnecessary trouble caused by your deepest desires. If you can learn to practice self-control, only acting when inspired and under the appropriate circumstances, you can prevent pain and suffering.

With my running, I learned this the hard way. At the beginning of 2025, I was eager to take my running to the next level. I added a day to my running schedule and tried to hit a goal of running an eight-minute mile. But in my excitement, I went too fast too soon and injured my calf muscle. The injury hurt so much that it not only kept me from running but also from walking. When I browsed videos on calf strain from running, they all said the same thing. A calf injury only happens when you increase your distance or speed too fast, and your muscles aren't ready to adapt. I now know that I have to take it slowly, no matter how much I want to get better and faster at running.

In the example of sexual desire, when you come together with another while holding the purpose of a blissful union, sex becomes a spiritual experience rather than a functional one. Or, when you eat something delicious, take the time to enjoy the process fully and eat only when hungry. Most modern people gobble down a meal at their desk or in their car while completing other tasks, never having the mindfulness toward sense control.

Blissfulness exists in waiting for the right moment or correct thought. Anyone can act impulsively on a desire or thought. But it takes a mature and skilled mind to sit back and act with discernment. That is the essence of brahmacharya.

☙ Living Brahmacharya off the Mat ❧

Practice discernment and have respect for your sexuality and creative force. The difference between humans and other animals is that humans have the power of discernment. You get to decide if you want to be wild and fancy-free or reserved and mindful. You have the power to delay pleasure or give in to it. That power is a gift that no other animal has. As an evolving yogi, use it toward union with your higher self or God. And as you "flow with Brahma" you'll know which actions to take when it comes to your creative life force.

☙ Practicing Brahmacharya on the Mat ❧

As you move on your yoga mat, practice loving every part of your body. Feel the creative flow move through you as you transition from one pose to another. While holding a pose, send love and happiness to the areas of your body you feel the most. Silently repeat, "I love you. I love you," to those parts.

For example, while holding *trikonasana*, triangle pose, feel into your feet, insoles, calves, and quads rising up into your hip sockets. Feel the expansion of your chest as it opens toward the sky and the extension of your arm and fingertips reaching for the heavens. Silently say, "Thank you," to the creative force pulsating through you, and thank each body part as it draws your attention to it.

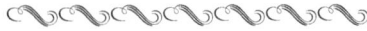

The 5th Yama

Aparigraha: Non-grasping, Detachment

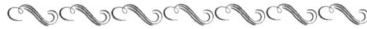

"When non-greed is confirmed, a thorough illumination of the how and why of one's birth comes."

—*Yoga Sutra 2.39*

Watching a toddler assert his freedom upon learning to run is one of the funniest and most exhilarating sights to behold. Once he finds that his legs can move faster than the slow pace of learning to walk, the toddler no longer walks but runs everywhere and at top speed. It's endearing to the observer of the grinning toddler, delighted with his newfound freedom but frustrating to the worried parent trying to reign in their wild child. When the chasing parent finally catches the wayward toddler, anger usually ensues. The frustrated parent clutches the child in anger, and the child screams in protest. Both are unhappy because this game of chase and catch feels wrong.

But the game is necessary for the child's safety, and if he's lucky, the child learns the lessons of safety through gentle parenting. However, the overly anxious parent who clings to their child throughout childhood will find him more rebellious, unhappy, or both since no one wants to be in the clutches of another.

Aparigraha teaches us that all of life works in this way. Nothing must be grasped or possessed as if it were only yours. In this physical existence, everything is temporary and ever-changing. You don't even get to hold onto your physical body. It changes and transforms from minute to minute. The body you had ten years ago is much different than the one you have today. And at the end of your life, you shed your human body because you can't take it with you.

I have a parent who hoards, which is the opposite of aparigraha. When I ask my mother why she keeps so many things, she responds, "I might need them one day." She also explains that her mother grew up during the Great Depression which influenced her to save everything as well. While hoarding is a mental health issue, the concept aligns with poverty consciousness. Poverty consciousness is based on fear and shows a lack of trust in the infinitely abundant universe.

Aparigraha calls you to trust in the nature of things. The birds do not worry about where they will find their next meal. They simply look and find it. Hoarding indicates that the universe has already given all it's going to give. In this mindset, you believe it's better to take yours before someone else does. In a way, this is similar to the third yama, *asteya*, or non-stealing.

People often look at their children, partners, and friends as possessions. They say things like "Don't look at my girlfriend," or "This is my best friend." In reality, we can never possess another person. We don't even own our children, although some try.

In his book *The Prophet*, the poet Kahlil Gibran wrote, "Your children are not your children. They are the sons and daughters of Life's longing for itself." In his parental wisdom, my dad always quoted that to me when raising my children.

Trying to hold onto things causes distress and unhappiness. When I hear my mom talking about "organizing her house," I cringe at the thought of the hours, days, weeks, months, and years spent trying to organize the millions of things in her house. If she could follow the wisdom of aparigraha, she would be liberated.

Many Americans have similar problems. They have so many things that they need to buy portable closets or pod storage sheds to store everything. Then, when those are overflowing, they rent space in a storage facility. It's silly when you think about it.

A Modern Take on Aparigraha

The concept of aparigraha helped the yogi assume a modest way of life. He would give up his worldly possessions to live in a forest academy or, centuries later, in an ashram. Depending on the guru he followed, he would give up everything except one robe and a bowl for begging.

This type of minimalist living is not desirable in most modern societies. Although some spiritual seekers might opt for the ancient yogic lifestyle, most are householders with modern jobs, families, and bills.

Like many religious teachings, the Yoga Sutras discourage lavish lifestyles. I even found verses suggesting one should feel shame for desiring wealth. For the modern yogi, I must emphasize that it's not shameful to want wealth. It all comes down to your character, intentions, and mindset.

Living Abundantly with an Aparigraha Mindset

In the opening paragraph, I stated that hoarding equaled a poverty mindset, which is true. But you are of the same mindset when you believe you must live minimally. To reiterate, filling your house with millions of things for fear that you might not have enough is poverty consciousness. Similarly, giving everything away and living with very little because you fear the rest of the world won't have enough is a lack mindset too.

The truth is you can't get poor enough to make one person rich on the planet. That isn't how wealth works. If you've ever been in a position where you couldn't pay your bills, it doesn't make you kind-hearted and humble. It makes you angry, scared, and frustrated. It also makes you despise others who can afford lavish dinners and drive around in new cars. Giving away everything you own is not the solution to happiness in modern times.

Our modern life calls for money and possessions. You mustn't feel shame or think you are less of a spiritual person for wanting the objects that make you feel like a complete person. The meaning behind aparigraha is about the attachment to those things.

I once dated a man in his early thirties who had acquired a lot of wealth by selling cryptocurrency. This man grew up in a family with hard-working parents. His parents were thrifty but sent him to private schools. They also frequented country clubs. While he and I got along fabulously, I was bothered by the fact that he was greedy with his money. Throughout the time we dated, he never bought me something as little as a cup of coffee. Every date came with a split check that he ensured the server knew about in advance. He would joke that his money was his and wouldn't spend it on anyone but himself. His attachment to money was one of the reasons we broke up. When a person has such an attachment to things, it feels wrong. You may know some people like this with money or other things like cars, motorcycles, or clothes.

While growing up, my mom would never let me touch the washer and dryer because she thought I might break them. So when I went to college, I didn't know I had to separate dark from light clothes, so I turned all my clothes pink.

When it came time to learn how to drive, I had to learn in our elderly neighbor's car because my mom wouldn't let me use hers. I wasn't allowed to use many of my mother's things, so I thought it was a general adult mindset. But, one summer, I was a nanny for a family with three kids. When they told me to use their car, I freaked out. My eyes widened, and I responded, "Wait, you want me to take your car?" The parents laughed and said, "Michelle, we're allowing you to watch our precious children all summer. Do you think it matters that we're letting you take our car?" That put things into perspective for me. Some people are more possessive of their objects than their children.

Having things is a part of modern life. We should enjoy our lives, and having things is part of that enjoyment. Yet, holding onto people and things for fear of losing them makes us unhappy.

The modern yogi must think in moderation. It's essential to let go of the fear of losing things. When you're not attached to things, you won't get devastated when you lose them or someone steals them.

Aparigraha in Modern Relationships

Clients come to me for intuitive guidance on their romantic relationships. Often, they're holding on to a person or relationship too tightly. Clutching or grasping a person you're dating or married to is the cause of many relationship problems. When you try to hold onto a romantic partner, you suffocate them. In grasping, you become controlling, and no one wants to be controlled.

Modern society teaches us that jealousy or showing possession is a sign of love. However, these ego-based traits only show selfish or conditional love. Conversely, practicing aparigraha in relationships helps foster unconditional love.

Non-Attachment

The concept of non-attachment is often misunderstood. Non-attachment means your world won't crumble if your object of attachment disappears. People frequently get too attached to people and things and can't recover when they lose them. But when you truly love from the point of non-attachment, you can say,

"I am still me. And that person is still themsevles. I have my autonomy, and they have theirs. We come together because we want to. And if we part ways, it's because we have other things to do in this lifetime. But whether we're together or apart, it doesn't change the fact that I am a whole person."

Embracing aparigraha in relationships causes you to love more and not less. As a whole and complete person who is an attractor of great things, you can love someone while not being dependent on them for love. When you come together because you both want to but don't need to, you experience bliss. In other words, love is magnified through non-attachment. But when you're attached and need the other person to be your source of love, you feel lifeless when they leave. Strive to find the love from your higher self first and allow love to flow in and out of your life with non-attachment.

Aparigraha with Objects and Identity

Dr. Wayne W. Dyer, used to say, "How do you experience water? You open your hand, stick it in, and allow the water to flow through." He would continue his analogy: "If you make a fist and try to grab at the water and say, 'come here water, let me get you,' you will never experience it."

Objects represent anything outside of yourself or an identity you establish to define yourself. For example, suppose you're a golfer. As a golfer, you buy the necessary items to play golf. You purchase high-end golf clubs, shoes, gloves, and a golf cart. In this scenario, you love your golf gear and believe the gear is what makes you a good golfer. What if, one day, someone breaks into your car and steals your golf clubs? Or worse, someone breaks into your garage and steals your golf cart, bag, and clubs? Would losing all the objects representing your golf game make you less of a golfer? I'm going to guess that while annoying, the loss of your golf gear would not make you a worse golfer. That is because all the skills you acquired while playing golf are still a part of you.

Here's a better example. What if you've spent decades accumulating wealth? Suppose you invest a million dollars into the stock market or a real estate project that tanks, causing you to lose all of it. Does that mean all is lost? While most people would feel depression and despair, the truth is that all is not lost. Motivational speaker Jim Rohn once said (and I am paraphrasing), "If you become a millionaire and lose it all, all is not lost. What it took to become a millionaire is still with you." That statement blew my mind when I first heard it. He was saying that all of the lessons, experiences, and knowledge gained in paving your way to a million dollars is still a part of you. Therefore, you can do it again and again and again. What better argument to not hoard the money you've made?

Finally, a lot of people identify themselves with their job or career. Often, this anchor is strong. Usually, when we meet someone, we ask them, "What do you do?" Or, "Where do you work?" Attachment to your job or career as a significant part of your identity can cause pain if you lose it or if it no longer satisfies you. In certain countries, some people commit suicide if they get fired because the attachment to that identity is so strong.

The longer we live, the more we realize that jobs and careers come and go. Many people reinvent themselves several times. Some of my favorite examples include Julia Childs, who became a master French chef at forty-nine; Louise Hay, who founded Hay House at sixty; and Laura Ingalls Wilder, who published her first *Little House on the Prairie* book at sixty-five. What if these women had stopped at their previous jobs or careers? We wouldn't have had the pleasure of their later-in-life creations.

How to Practice Non-Attachment

The best way to practice non-attachment is to consider yourself the director of your life. In this, you might say things like:

- *I am not my body, but I have a body.*
- *I am not my emotions, but I have emotions.*
- *I am not my job, but I have a job.*

In other words, you begin to see the roles you play without being attached to them.

Suppose you're a mom and identify strongly with this role. During the week, you work as a financial consultant. While working, you speak to your co-workers and boss in your best mom voice. "Did you wash your hands after going to the bathroom?" "Here, your nose is running; let me wipe it for you." "You look tired. Go lie down and take a nap immediately." You're laughing, perhaps. But if you did that, they might haul you off for a mental health evaluation. In this example, assuming you must play the mom in every situation sounds ridiculous. And yet, how many parents go into a deep depression when their children leave home? It's just as silly.

When you can step back and declare that you have things to play with, people with whom to play, and roles to enjoy, your life is happier, healthier, and whole. In this relaxed state of aparigraha, things come and go like the ebb and flow of the ocean's tides. In this state, you begin to trust that when objects and people come in, they're meant to come in, and when they leave, they're meant to go. In this mindset, you are always in a state of peace.

Interpretation of the Yoga Sutra 2-39

When non-greed is confirmed, a thorough illumination of the how and why of one's birth comes. -Yoga Sutra 2-39

The threads of the Yoga Sutras point you toward the realization of your true nature. Before you came here, you had pure potential and were the source of unconditional love. As you incarnated into your human form, you kept a portion of your eternal essence. In other words, you agreed to come here and complete certain tasks but never intended to completely forget your infinite nature.

Attachment or greed, as put in the Yoga Sutra, is a byproduct of the human condition. As humans, we need a lot. We need air, food, water, shelter, and good immune systems to fight off germs. We need others to help us navigate life. And we need them for love and connection. This neediness causes us to grasp people and things. But it also causes worry, anxiety, and fear. So, by letting go of the worry, anxiety, and fear, you also let go of attachment and begin to trust in your true nature. Your true nature is the God or Universal Source part of you.

You never intended to starve or be deprived of what you need for this earthly journey. Before you came, you set the intention to have everything you would need. When you practice aparigraha, you are illuminated to this truth. In this knowing, you relax. And the more you relax, knowing that you have everything you need for this journey, the more you begin to trust in the oneness that is you.

❧ Living Aparigraha off the Mat ❧

Practice living aparigraha off the mat with the following exercises and affirmations.

1. I will notice feelings of jealousy or envy and remind myself that no one can take what is mine if it's needed for my journey.
2. I will remind myself that everyone has the freedom to be who they are in every moment, in-

cluding myself. When I start to feel possessive of another person, I will ponder unconditional love and adjust my thoughts to the ebb and flow of life.

3. I will realize that sharing my things, including money, with others is easy because goodness continuously flows to me.

4. When I get angry or upset about someone taking my parking space or cutting in front of me at the grocery store, I'll pause and realize there is enough for everyone. I will remind myself that infinite abundance is everywhere.

Practicing Aparigraha on the Mat

When you arrive for your mat practice, come with zero expectations. Be open to immersing yourself fully into the experience. Holding onto expectations of having a particular yoga teacher, a specific spot, the room's temperature, or performing certain yoga poses during class can make you unhappy if those desires are unmet. Instead, come into class with the attitude: *I will allow goodness to be a part of my experience today.* You are guaranteed a good class when you begin your yoga asana practice with this mindset.

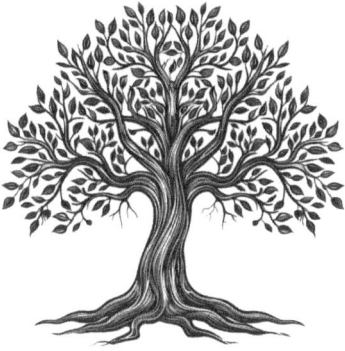

CHAPTER 2

The 2nd Limb of Yoga

The Niyamas

Niyama consists of purity, contentment, intense discipline, the study of spiritual books for self-understanding, and surrender to God (Self). —Yoga Sutra 2.32

The second limb of yoga outlines personal observances. The niyamas include *shoucha*: purity, *santosha*: contentment, *tapas*: discipline, *svadhyaya*: spiritual study or self-study, and *ishwara-pranidhana*: surrender to the divine.

The niyamas build upon one another to prepare a yoga student for the intense demands of asana and pranayama.

Sometimes, when we see a list of rules, we want to avoid them. We may find them too constricting and fear losing our freedom. But as you will see, when following the yamas and niyamas, the rewards become apparent with consistent practice.

Here's how it works. You will feel better and better as you purify your body and mind. In your contentment, you are compelled to stick with the process of keeping your body and mind clear of toxins. As you observe the changes within you, you will begin to notice your shortcomings and wish to transform them. With your new habits, you'll want to study more yoga and learn more about living a yoga lifestyle. Living a yoga lifestyle makes you less concerned with your daily problems. You will brush off obstacles as minor annoyances that will work themselves out. Because of your yoga practice, you will come to believe in the power of your higher spiritual self and universal Source. Therefore, your life will flow effortlessly, and you'll experience fewer problems and more joy.

In reading that paragraph, did you feel the stress of following rules or the liberation of a happier and more fulfilling life? With practice, you'll move toward a more purposeful and fulfilling life and away from a stressful one.

Patanjali wrote the niyamas for those living in an ashram where deep yoga study was a daily devotion. However, students seeking enlightenment weren't punished for not following these guidelines; they were encouraged to look within and practice more mindfully.

According to The Upanishads, connecting with your higher self brings you more joy.

The Self is the source of abiding joy. Our hearts are filled with joy in seeing him. Enshrined in the depths of our consciousness. If he were not there, who would breathe, who live? He is the one who fills every heart with joy.-
The Taittiriya Upanishad, Part II, 7-1

Each practice helps you uncover the layers of your hidden Self; as you etch away at the excess, you begin to see your true nature.

CRCRCRCRCR

The 1st Niyama

Shoucha: Purity

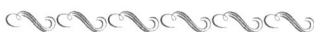

CRCRCRCR

With bodily purification, you recoil from the body and disassociate from others. —Yoga Sutra 2.40

Purification also brings about clarity, happiness, concentration, mastery of the senses, and capacity for self-awareness— Yoga Sutra 2.41

In reading four different interpretations of shoucha, I'm astonished that the interpreters, all men, have gotten this niyama so far off course. The purpose of the first five limbs of yoga is to get the practitioner to the point of forgetting about the physical body and its constant demands. So, when you meditate, your body isn't bothering you. As I've mentioned, the end goal of the Eight Limbs of Yoga is to find union with the Self. And it's challenging to do that while your body asks for things like food, water, sleep, pain relief, etc.

Every interpretation I've seen of shoucha points to the body as a disgusting thing that must be ignored. Additionally, these interpretations state that physical touch with another must be avoided entirely. According to The Upanishads, *The Hatha Yoga Pradipika*, and the Yoga Sutras, these interpretations are wrong. I believe these interpretations were convenient for life in ashrams or forest academies. It makes sense. In teaching pubescent boys, it may have been necessary to encourage cleanliness. It may also have been essential to tell the boys to stop touching themselves and others. Then, throughout time, this became the interpretation of shoucha. However, the texts mentioned above tell a different story.

In *The Hatha Yoga Pradipika*, body purification is emphasized as a ritual practice before engaging in asana and pranayama. These practices, such as *neti*: nasal wash, *nauli*: stomach cleanse, and *basti*: herbal enema, help clear toxins to open the circulatory channels for prana to flow during yoga asana and pranayama. This is a more accurate description of shoucha.

In modern times, many are disconnected from their bodies, but not in a way a yogi might be who has attained purity through practice. For example, modern people overeat and eat foods laden with sugar, fat, and chemicals. Many drink alcohol excessively, smoke nicotine or marijuana regularly, or take drugs. Additionally, a sedentary lifestyle doesn't allow the body to purge toxins daily. Therefore, forgetting about the body isn't exactly the goal for a modern yogi until they have reached the point of habitual disciplinary practice.

Physical purity

Fasting, dieting, and detoxes are popular in modern life. If you follow fads, you'll constantly find something new related to all three. Yet, a yogic way of life encourages constant bodily care, with a vegetarian diet and eating only two meals daily. Modern society has cutting-edge supplements, powders, and herbs to help a person detox. But most people I know go back to a lifestyle of sugar, fatty and fried foods, lots of meat, and alcohol after a three or seven-day fast or detox. According to physical purity, a yogi must follow healthy eating daily with occasional treats, and not the opposite. A healthy diet should be the norm.

Additionally, modern life requires us to spend a lot of time indoors, where the air is stale or recycled and we have little exposure to the benefits of sunlight. If you live in a city, you might be affected by smog or other pollutants. The healing effects of fresh air, sunlight, and natural elements also help purify the body.

Finally, exercise is essential. One of the body purification techniques mentioned in *The Hatha Yoga Pradipika*, also a *panchakarma* technique in Ayurveda, is svedana, or sweating. The body must sweat to rid itself of toxins. Generally, if you aren't moving your body, you're not sweating. Another modern invention, air conditioning, can cause us to avoid sweating altogether. In the chapter on the fourth limb of yoga, pranayama, I'll give more details on detoxification and opening the body's channels.

Mental purity

In modern times, we're stuck in a mental stress-fest. Toxins that build up from social media, the news, text messages, and emails are real. You know firsthand that the constant demands for your attention can bring you mental anguish. In addition, societal expectations can lead to excessive mental stress, especially from social media, where people can appear to have a perfect life or body.

You've likely heard the term "social media detox." I would take it one step further and encourage you to detox from the news and current events. Mental purity means don't focus on negativity or obsessive thoughts. When your attention is on adverse events beyond your control, you take in a lot of negativity. Then, life appears more gloomy than it is.

Perhaps you've also heard the phrase; *Comparison is the thief of joy?* A lot of social media is either about complaining or comparison. As you desire a cleaner mental space, you will notice that conversations and chatter on social media will bother you more and more. When you reach that point, you will know it's time to focus on more fulfilling topics.

Spiritual purity

Your spiritual connection can't remain pure if you're stuck on your mental or intellectual faculties. As a human being having a spiritual experience, you will always swing back and forth from your humanness to your God-self. You are never quite one or the other, but both. Since your conception, you've always had a direct connection with Source. Dr. Wayne W. Dyer used to say, "But how rusty is the link?" In other words, we and others tend to corrode the link with belief systems, self-imposed limitations, rules, and regulations.

You must understand that you are already pure. Modern religion wouldn't have you believe that, but it's true. You are pure. Your body is pure. Your mind is pure. And your soul is pure. But, if you've been hard on yourself because you're not the perfect yogi or the perfect human being, you corrode the link connecting you to God.

You can clean up the connection between you and your Higher Source by giving yourself grace and connecting with your spiritual self daily.

Living Shoucha off the Mat

When practicing shoucha off the mat, you pay closer attention to what you put into your body and mind and what goes out. For example, do you have purity of speech, or do you like to gossip? Do you have purity of mind? Or do you enjoy competing with and getting ahead of others, even at their expense? Do you have addictions that keep you rooted in excess? Ponder these daily and make changes when it's appropriate to make them.

⤷ Practicing Shoucha on the Mat ⤶

As you enter a yoga class and begin your asana practice, observe your body and mind. A pure pose is one in which your only goal is improving your practice. For example, focus on yourself instead of showing others or the instructor that you can get into a perfect pose. Even if you can do the pose better than others, know you're only competing with yourself.

Purity also includes not judging others for their body shape, size, fitness level, or what they might be wearing. It means you spend your yoga time focusing on yourself and your well-being. Your time is well-spent when you cease to compare or judge others or yourself and observe a more wholesome asana practice.

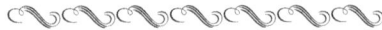

∽∾∽∾∽∾∽∾∽∾∽∾

The 2nd Niyama

Santosha: Contentment

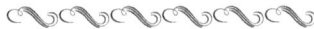

∽∾∽∾∽∾∽∾∽∾

From contentment, supreme joy is gained.

—*Yoga Sutra 2.42*

In the Law of Attraction, it is evident that the one central principle in attaining all that you desire is contentment. While I'm not new to the principles of manifestation and co-creation, I recently discovered the teachings of Abraham through Esther Hicks. In a You-

Tube video that Esther and Jerry Hicks posted in 2012, they played a theme song with the refrain, "Joy is the key." If you've had the pleasure of listening to any or all of the Abraham recordings, it's easy to whittle down the messages into one word: joy.

Joy, contentment, or satisfaction are ways to feel enlightened every second of every day. Another word closely related to joy is bliss, or, in Sanskrit, *ananda*. Joy and bliss are different from the concept of happiness. Happiness usually depends on an external factor, such as having money, the right job, or finding a lover. Joy, or *sukha* in Sanskrit, is long-lasting and independent of external factors. Therefore, happiness is transient, while joy is everlasting.

Here, the Yoga Sutra explains that the pathway to joy is through the practice of contentment.

The Practice of Contentment

The other day, I posted a dresser for sale on the social media site NextDoor. I'm not a fan of this site because people use this platform to complain. Although it's not the only thing that happens, it's the predominant theme. Usually, the person who complains uses the platform to attract sympathizers, and it becomes a "misery loves company" scenario.

Just like complaining, practicing contentment is a habit. Given a choice, contentment is the better choice. With so many variations of things to focus on, choosing what makes you feel good and satisfied will take you much further on your spiritual path.

When my son got into an accident that totaled his car, I thought things were terrible. And they were. While my son was completely fine, many unpleasant things needed to be done to get him up and running again. Additionally, the cost involved nearly depleted his savings. After we caught our breath the next day, I looked at him and stated, "This sucks. But from here on out, everyone we engage with throughout this process will be helpful and pleasant." And that statement became a reality. We both knew the only thing that really mattered was his health and well-being. And we also knew that our attitude would determine the outcome of these unpleasant tasks. Our contentment for his well-being allowed us to see the blessings with every person we encountered. As a result, people went out of their way to help us. Even the insurance company valued the car at $3,000 above what we thought they might. Contentment brought us joy in what we thought to be a joyless situation.

It's easy to practice contentment when events and circumstances are going your way. It's much more difficult to practice when your life seems to be falling apart.

Everything Has Two Sides

During the worldwide pandemic, we saw the dichotomy of life. For example, if you had to work outside the home five days per week, put your kids in daycare, and had a long daily commute, you saw the complete opposite in 2020. In the blink of an eye, you were working at home, the kids were virtually attending school, and you weren't allowed to go out. If you thrived in your previous life, staying at home was punishment. But if you hated the stress of your life before March 2020, you felt blessed.

Here's another example. Before the pandemic, perhaps there were times you hated going out to get food, especially on a cold winter's day. But after a year of quarantine, you probably jumped at the first opportunity to go out to eat, even in the dead of winter.

It is essential to gain perspective on choosing contentment versus dissatisfaction. Since everything has two sides, it's impossible to know if a situation will improve or hinder your life.

I first read the following Zen Buddhist story in a children's picture book, *Zen Shorts*, by Jon J. Muth. I've taken the liberty of paraphrasing a version of the story. Within a few lines, you'll understand how events are more pliable than you've been led to believe.

A long time ago, there was a poor farmer whose only horse ran away. His neighbors told him, "How unfortunate that your horse ran away. You are so unlucky." The farmer responded, "Maybe. We shall see."

The next day, the horse came back with a beautiful mare. His neighbors told him, "How fortunate. Your luck has turned." The farmer responded, "We shall see."

A week later, the farmer's son mounted the mare to tame it. The horse bucked him, and he broke his leg.

The neighbors told the farmer, "Your son has broken his leg. Your new mare is a curse." The farmer responded, "We shall see."

The following month, the army came to recruit all first-born sons to war. Since the farmer's son's leg was still broken, they didn't take him. His neighbors cried, "You are so lucky!" The farmer responded. "We shall see."

The moral of the story is that we can never know, with any degree of certainty, whether something is good or bad. If you choose contentment, you will see the silver lining in every situation.

Gratitude to Counteract the Reptilian Brain

You've probably noticed that your brain skews negative. I opened this section with a story about the site NextDoor and the negativity of its users. The reason complaining is so prevalent is because of the reptilian portion of the brain. The same region responsible for the fight-flight-freeze response is the survivalist part, the amygdala. The prefrontal cortex, responsible for judgment and higher-level thinking, is more recently developed and requires more conscious thought. In instantaneous reactions, the amygdala often takes over. That is why negative headlines and news are so attractive to most; we want to know how to survive at all times.

Since the survival instinct is rooted in fear, one way to counter the fear is with gratitude, which leads to contentment. The concept of gratitude may seem overused. It can feel too simplistic. But it works. Here's why: you can't hold a feeling of gratitude and fear simultaneously. It's impossible.

Try this exercise. Place your awareness on the following phrases. Read them each three times.

1. I am grateful for the air I breathe and all the fresh air.
2. I am grateful for the sun, sky, clouds, rain, and wind.
3. I am grateful for the moon, stars, night sky, and planetary bodies.
4. I am grateful for my body, including my heart, lungs, intestines, skin, hands, arms, shoulders, chest, legs, knees, feet, and ankles...
5. I am grateful for my home.
6. I am grateful for the people I love and who love me.
7. I am grateful for the food I have now and have had.
8. I am grateful for clean water.
9. I am grateful for the grass, trees, plants, and flowers.
10. I am grateful for the animals on the planet.
11. I am grateful for the oceans, streams, rivers, ponds, and all other bodies of water.
12. I am grateful for life.

How do you feel after reading the list three times? Even though it wasn't nearly exhaustive with everything you can be grateful for in each moment, do you feel a little more upbeat?

The best thing about an exercise like the one above is that once you gain momentum, you want to keep going. If you choose to keep the positive momentum going, you will experience more joy daily.

☙ Living Santosha off the Mat ❧

Practicing present-moment awareness is the key to living santosha off the mat. When rooted in the present moment, focus on what is here now. Then, it will be easier to remain in a state of gratitude. We usually perceive situations, circumstances, and events as problems because we choose to live in the past or project into an imaginary future. But when you stop the flow of thought to the past or future, you notice the beauty of your present circumstances. Even if your present situation is not ideal, appreciate the good things. Appreciation will lead to contentment. In searching for positive aspects of a person or situation, you will continue to find more positive ones. Once you gain momentum, your contentment will continue to grow.

☙ Practicing Santosha on the Mat ❧

Hold gratitude and contentment for each body part during the pose. Even when feeling muscle tension or discomfort, thank your body for warning you that something isn't quite right. Throughout the day, our bodies give us signals that we tend to ignore. Then, when we reach our beds, we say, "Oh, my back hurts so much!" Or, "I have a headache the size of Mount Everest!" The gentle prods your body gives are signals to readjust or realign. Thank your body for talking to you, and honor it by adjusting your pose during a yoga session to accommodate it.

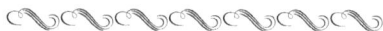

❧❧❧❧❧❧

The 3rd Niyama

Tapas: Discipline

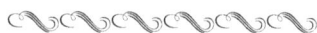

❧❧❧❧❧

Impurities are destroyed by austerity (discipline), and the body and senses become refined.

—Yoga Sutra 2.43

Six days a week, I wake up at 5:20 a.m. to drink a mocha, do my personal hygiene routine, meditate, and head to the gym for an intense workout. No one makes me do this. I'm self-employed and have been for many years. I have this rigid routine because it makes me feel good. I feel productive and accomplished as I start my day. Even if nothing else gets done, I know I've started my day well.

While we are creatures of habit, discipline hasn't been widely practiced in the past decade. Modern life has made people lazy and complacent. For example, many don't make the effort anymore, as wardrobe requirements for work and social engagements have become less stringent. Teenagers attend school in pajamas and slippers, and many adults don't wear much more than jeans and a T-shirt, even in social situations. As an overwhelmed mom of three young kids, I had difficulty cleaning and organizing my home. The more I did, the more I had to do. Toys were everywhere. And every piece of rug or furniture had foodstuff embedded in it. I always felt I was behind and was in a constant state of despair. I wanted to enjoy my kids, but instead, I worried constantly about my to-do list. One day, a friend sent me an email that changed my life. She had discovered Marla Cilley, also known as The Fly Lady. Marla's instructions for a better life were simple. Get up in the morning, get dressed, and put on your shoes with laces. The next step is to shine your kitchen sink. It sounds trivial. But it worked! Discipline helps to unravel the chaos in your body, mind, and environment.

A yogi is disciplined. Everything about a yoga lifestyle trains your body, mind, and emotions into habitual practices that become automatic. The word *tapas* in Sanskrit means "fire." Fire burns and transforms. Your disciplinary practices will mold you into a better version of yourself through their transformative nature.

Athletes know this firsthand. Take, for example, basketball player Larry Bird. Since high school, he began every day with 500 jump shots. He also challenged himself to hit 99 free throws in a row. And if he didn't do it, he would start again.[4]

Many believe that people become successful or famous out of luck. While luck can be a factor, 99% of all successful people live a disciplined lifestyle. Author

Malcolm Gladwell asserted in his book *Outliers* that mastery is achieved with talent plus preparation. The preparation part of the equation equals 10,000 hours of practice on a given task before a person sees great success.[5] One of the reasons yoga students stayed in the forest academies for up to twelve years was so they could master the yogic principles.

Living a disciplined lifestyle is also soothing because most humans love routines. It's usually when doing a mundane task such as emptying the dishwasher or folding laundry that you get a brilliant idea.

Furthermore, through the process of repetition, you get better. As Tony Robbins' mentor, Jim Rohn, taught, "Repetition is the mother of skill." Even if you do sun salutations daily, you can always find a way to realign or relax into each pose.

Understandably, not everyone who embarks upon a yogic journey wants to achieve mastery or become a yoga teacher. However, most begin yoga to get relief from physical or emotional ailments. In our quick-fix society, many want an immediate cure. The mantra becomes, Give me a pill, machine, or hack that will fix me fast. But yoga is not a hack.

Most students will get some relief from one yoga class. But since yoga is a lifestyle and not a sixty or ninety-minute cure-all, the ailments will resurface. Daily practice, repetition, and integration will work to reduce symptoms and keep illness at bay.

The second part of the Yoga Sutra explains, "Your body and senses become refined." With daily practice, your intuition will guide you to stand and stretch or take a couple of minutes to do pranayama. In other words, you can better tune into your body and senses to understand exactly what you need at any moment because you will be reconnected.

❧ Living Tapas off the Mat ☙

It's easy to run from a disciplined lifestyle because the word discipline reminds us of school, parents, or the law. Confinement, restrictions, and limitations are other words that come to mind with discipline. Yuck! Right? But have you ever set the intention to start an exercise regime? While it was difficult to start, after the first workout, you probably felt amazing. The more you create healthy and helpful routines and habits, the more you want to do them. After a while, it doesn't feel like work at all; it feels exciting. Strive for feelings of excitement and enthusiasm when approaching your disciplined practices. Instead of saying, "I have to do…" Say, "I get to do this! Yes!"

❧ Practicing Tapas on the Mat ☙

Author James Clear, in his book *Atomic Habits*, explains that you can build a habit by doing it for just one or two minutes per day. If you want to start a daily yoga practice, have your mat set up before you go to bed. On the first day, do one minute of yoga asanas; the next day, do two minutes, and so on. To have a disciplined practice, consistency is key. Often, people tend to have an all-or-nothing approach when building a habit, and they quit before starting. Set realistic expectations for yourself by starting small.

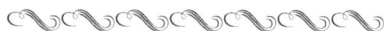

❦❦❦❦❦❦❦

The 4th Niyama

Svadhyaya: Spiritual or Self-Study

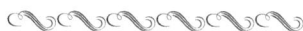

❦❦❦❦❦

Self-study and introspection deepen communion with the Divine.

-Yoga Sutra 2.44

We are living in a time of deep psychology. Now, more than ever, people are turning to psychological concepts such as Attachment Theory, inner child wounds, co-dependency, boundary setting, and studying various forms of the Myers-Briggs personality types and astrology. People are becoming more self-aware. They want to know more about themselves. And that is a good thing.

Traditionally, *svadhyaya* was translated to mean "the study of spiritual literature." As a serious yoga student, you would study The Bhagavad Gita, The Upanishads, and The Vedas. You can certainly reap benefits from studying spiritual texts. I had an uplifting experience the first time I read The Upanishads. However, it's not required to connect with your spiritual self.

Some authors translate svadhyaya to mean Self-study, meaning the inward journey. Looking inward helps you understand what might be keeping you from recognizing your higher self.

Spiritual Texts

Through years of spiritual study, I've realized that all spiritual texts, while inspired by God, are channeled through humans. In other words, the person receiving the spiritual messages has a mind, intellect, ego, personality, and emotions. Their memories come from their emotional reactions to the events they've experienced. Throughout time, spiritual teachers have heard divine messages at different levels of awareness. So, you can never know if a channeled message is pure. For a message to be pure, the channel must also be pure, which isn't always the case.

Suppose you're a spiritual teacher having a bad day. On that day, when receiving divine messages, you might filter them through your bad mood. As a result, the transmission of pure light has been dimmed by your lower frequency. Most people don't take this into account when reading ancient spiritual literature.

All spiritual texts have validity and truth. The resonance with God-consciousness comes through them, and that's why many have withstood the test of time. But we don't consider the messengers' humanness in our search for divine perfection. Furthermore, many ancient texts have been translated time and again from the original language, so words and meanings get lost in translation. Finally, it isn't easy to know with certainty the meaning and context at the time the texts were written.

So, instead of taking spiritual texts at face value word by word, it's essential to be discerning and receive the general meaning rather than the specifics. And that brings us to the value or lack thereof of religion.

Religious Study

A few years ago, I went to a Christmas Eve mass at a catholic church with my mom. I was raised catholic but hadn't been to a catholic church for years. As I listened to the priest give his sermon, I found it endearing and innocent. I didn't think of it condescendingly but rather how a twelve-grade teacher would look at a kindergarten teacher teaching her students. It felt elementary. I've awakened to many spiritual truths over the past twenty-five years; therefore, catholic teachings appear to be child's play.

Today, I consider religious study to be similar to training wheels. Religion, rich in history, is part of our human story. To deny its validity would be foolish. Every society has its form of religion because we have an innate desire to commune with our souls. If religion were an anomaly, we wouldn't see the perpetual birth and rebirth of religious organizations. Religions are microcosms of societies. They give us guidance, rules, morality, community, commonality, education, and spirituality. They fulfill the need for inclusion, service to humanity, and love and connection. It's no wonder the expansion of religious organizations has been a constant.

However, religions are limited. For those seeking an extension of society with a splash of God, they can fulfill that purpose. But they fail for the serious spiritual student seeking a personal and transcendent experience.

When an organization implies that you must turn to a religious or spiritual leader to provide you with the knowledge and experience of God, it cuts you short of self-realization. But when an organization or teacher says, "You don't need me, turn to your Source." That is when you know you've reached an enlightened being. An enlightened teacher will never point to themselves as the source of knowledge; they will always direct you back to yourself.

That is why religion is a starting point. A good religious organization will give you the template to follow until you're focused enough to follow your own path. However, most people aren't curious enough to go off alone. They will remain with their training wheels for fear of falling.

Study Inspirational Texts

After suggesting that the pathway to self-realization is the only way, it may seem counterintuitive to encourage the study of inspirational and spiritual texts. However, reading about those who have arrived at the place you wish to be can help you get there. Sometimes, all it takes is one phrase, quote, or idea to propel you forward. I spent years studying inspirational and spiritual material before I began teaching.

Infusing yourself with the written word helps you transcend. In addition, the more time you spend on spiritual and inspirational material, the less time you will spend on mindless activities such as TV watching, internet surfing, or social media browsing. Finally, as you read books from authors who have had a spiritual shift toward oneness, your vibration shifts as you read them.

❧ Living Svadhyaya off the Mat ❧

Become the observer of your thoughts, words, and actions. When I teach meditation, I speak about the observer and the observed. You can see your choices in each moment as you observe yourself going through daily life without judgment. This self-study can lead you to make better choices. For example, if you want to criticize a friend for being late, your observer (higher self) can internally reason: *I will show some compassion. I don't know why she was late. Perhaps I could ask rather than assume poor intentions.* The more you observe and study yourself, the more you move from separateness to oneness.

❧ Practicing Svadhyaya on the Mat ❧

Dedicate your yoga asana practice to an area of spiritual study. For example, one week, you could dedicate your practice to ahimsa. You could dedicate the following week to santosha, etc. I've done different spiritual studies on the mat. I was trained in the *Seven Spiritual Laws of Yoga* from Dr. Deepak Chopra's book, *The Seven Spiritual Laws of Success*. Over seven weeks, I taught and practiced one of the spiritual laws. I've also done the same with the seven chakras and wrote about it in my book, *Chakra Healing for Vibrant Energy*. Coupling your spiritual study with movement is a great way to learn and absorb it.

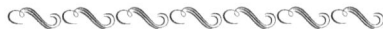

Cℛℛℛℛℛℛℛ

The 5th Niyama

Ishwara Pranidhana: Surrender to the Divine

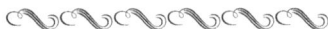

Cℛℛℛℛℛℛ

By total surrender to God, samadhi is attained.

—*Yoga Sutra 2.45*

The first two words defining the word surrender are cease resistance. These words perfectly explain the meaning in this context. *Ishwara* means God. And *pranidhana* indicates "from total surrender" or "from placing before." In other words, you reach total union when you place God first.

The concept of surrender can evoke negative feelings in those who are scarred by their religious upbringing. In many contexts, surrender indicates defeat or weakness. In the yogic spiritual context, however, surrender means releasing resistance.

In our separateness from Source, ourselves, and each other, we seek control. We strive to make things happen, take the bull by the horns, and force our lives into submission. Then, we get upset when life doesn't go our way.

By surrendering to God and your higher self, you admit that you can't control people, circumstances, and events into being precisely what you want. In this mindset, you move with universal force instead of pushing against it. You will still get what you want by going with the flow, but it will become much easier as you allow the universe to work with you.

Along with surrender comes the word trust. You learn to trust that things will always work out for you. With this trust or faith, you don't need to know how things will come together; you just know they will.

Many people look at surrender as a weakness. They think submission to God means having no power. That is because their concept of God is skewed. They believe that God is a judge, punisher, or stern parent. But submitting to that divine force would always be beneficial if they could see the truth that God is unconditional love. If you are working in concert with a Being who loves you unconditionally, there is no limit to what you can accomplish.

Submitting to Unconditional Love

In 2005, I was reading Dr. Deepak Chopra's book, *The Spontaneous Fulfillment of Desire.* An exercise in the book helps you discover your life's purpose with one simple question: *Why are you here?* The exercise instructs you to ask yourself the question twenty-five times in a row. Initially, I had various answers, such as, "I am here to write books." "I'm here to be a mom." But by the time I reached number fifteen, the answer was the same: "I am here to serve God." Nothing else came through.

If you have pain from your religious upbringing, try replacing the word "God" with something that represents God. For example, you could say, "I am here to serve unconditional love." Or, "I am here in service of joy." It doesn't matter how you word it; the concept is the same.

As you live in accordance with unconditional love, you no longer second-guess kind acts. For example, if you see a homeless person, your compassion might compel you to reach for five dollars. But sometimes, your mind kicks in with judgments: *Well, if I give him the five dollars, he's probably going to spend it on alcohol or drugs.* Living in service to God and unconditional love means you give the five dollars if you feel compelled to give. As Mother Theresa taught, "It's not between you and them. It's between you and God."

Oneness Is the End Goal

The second half of the Yoga Sutra states, "samadhi is attained." What is samadhi? It is oneness. When you serve God and, by extension, humanity, you feel at one with others.

Surrendering to the ego would be the opposite. When you surrender to your ego, you believe you are separate. Your mind goes to thoughts like, *I better get mine before someone else does. Or, That person hurt me, so I'm going to withhold love from them.* Source never thinks like that toward you or anyone else. Imagine if Source said one day, *Humans haven't been good today. I think I'll get rid of all the oxygen.* It sounds extreme, and yet we do this to one another.

Surrendering to God leads you to freedom. You will be free from the confines of the ego and its limitations. And your pathway to joy will become more prominent. The Shevatashvatara Upanishad says, "Wake up from this dream of separateness." This concept of unity is prevalent in all the Upanishads.

When one realizes the Self, in whom all life is one, changeless, nameless, formless, one fears no more. Until we realize the unity of life, we live in fear.

—*The Taittiriya Upanishad 7.1*

The ego equals fear, while the higher self equals love. Strive to live through the Self by submitting to it, and fear will be a distant memory.

Living Ishwara Pranidhana off the Mat

In your daily life, practice accepting what is. Most people spend so much time resisting and fighting against what is, that they wind up tired and frustrated. Accepting what is doesn't mean you won't want to change things. It means you'll find a way to release resistance when you don't have any control over a situation. For example, you could get upset if you go to the post office to mail a package and see a long line with one worker behind the counter. You could have a whole narrative about how inefficient post offices are and their inability to hire more employees or work faster. But that would make your experience unpleasant. Instead, you could surrender to standing in line by noticing human interactions, such as a smile when someone holds the door for someone else. Or, you could listen to a podcast or video while waiting. You could even strike up a conversation. Surrendering to the things you can't control gives you more choices to improve your life experiences.

In recovery circles, *The Serenity Prayer* outlines surrender:

God, grant me the serenity to accept the things I cannot change,

The courage to change the things I can,

And the wisdom to know the difference.

Applying these three simple lines can make a huge difference in your daily life.

⌒ Practicing Ishwara Pranidhana on the Mat

Surrender to your body today. Your body has an innate wisdom in connection with your higher self. It knows what is right for you at every moment. Tune into its inner knowing and honor what it needs. For example, if you go to yoga intending to get into a headstand, but your body isn't ready, you could injure yourself if you fail to surrender. Yogic surrender means releasing resistance. If your body wants a few more minutes of child's pose, surrender to it. And if your body needs a power yoga class, surrender to that. The more you surrender to your body, the faster you'll see progress.

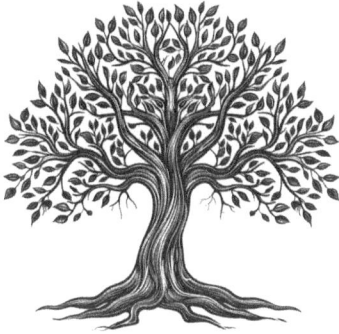

CHAPTER 3

The 3rd Limb of Yoga

Asana

Asana is a steady, comfortable posture.

—-Yoga sutra 2.46

After my first yoga class in 1989, I became a yoga purest. I studied hatha yoga, pranayama, and meditation. I would only accept the meditative type of yoga that a hatha yoga practice provides. So, as I took classes with different teachers throughout the years, I was turned off by those who didn't adhere to the type of yoga I was accustomed to. Doing vinyasa or kundalini yoga at the time didn't feel good, so I refrained. Yet, as the years passed, I began to appreciate and teach other styles.

In truth, there isn't a right or wrong type of yoga asana practice. The first Yoga Sutra states, "Asana is a steady, comfortable posture." When I see students performing advanced twists, turns, and acrobatics, I know those variations of asana aren't for me. They don't feel comfortable to me, but they might to those performing them.

I also used to have strong opinions about why people take yoga. As yoga became popular in the United States, I saw many treat it as another fitness class instead of a sacred spiritual practice. This wasn't easy to see since yoga had always been a sacred practice for me. However, as I expanded my yoga teaching into vinyasa and power yoga, I realized that yoga practitioners can still benefit from the spiritual aspects of yoga while getting fit.

That being said, asana ceases to be beneficial when you're disconnected from your body and push it to do things it's not ready to do. That's when you can get injured. Focusing on the true meaning of yoga, union, while practicing postures will teach you to listen to and flow with your body.

If you were to observe me taking a yoga class, you would see me in the back corner doing something different from the rest of the class. Sometimes, I follow the teacher but change variations every few breaths to honor my body. I learned this through years of taking yoga but mastered it in 2008 with my master teacher, Claire Diab, who led my yoga teacher training at the Chopra Center.

At the time of my training, Claire had been teaching yoga for over twenty years. When she started, she was told she could never earn a living teaching yoga. However, she proved everyone wrong. To make a living as a full-time yoga teacher, she taught twenty-three weekly classes in every scenario possible. At first, she had been trained in the Iyengar method with blocks, bolsters, and straps to help her students reach a perfect pose. After a while, tired of the cerebral, precision-based teaching, she decided to teach a class based on how her body felt. She explained that the first class she taught using her intuition and body's wisdom was liberating and more authentic than any class she had previously taught. She formed her style of flow with aspects of Qi Gong, which I still practice today.

Additionally, Claire starts her class by stating, "If you need to lie in savasana, relaxation pose, for the entire class, then do it. Honor your body." As the Yoga Sutra states, her classes were not difficult but steady and comfortable.

Communion with Your Body

Whether you take a yoga class or teach, your asana practice is about communion with your body. You will feel dissatisfied if you're not in alignment while practicing asana.

In modern living, we're taught, from an early age, that we must follow our teachers. We're taught to sit in our chairs, stay in one place, and follow everything our teacher tells us to do. Then, when we become adults, we still follow this indoctrination. Observe your next yoga class, and you will find this to be true. If you have a mix of young and old students in the same class, some are not ready for the complex poses a teacher might present. And yet, even in their unreadiness, you see them over-stretching, over-articulating their joints, and having painful looks on their faces while holding a pose. They want to follow the teacher and class so badly that they ignore how their body feels.

A great yoga teacher will present four or five variations of every pose. An expert teacher will return to the beginning variation after presenting the most complicated form of the pose. Here's why: since we are so accustomed to following the teacher, we will feel uneasy and out of place if we perform the beginner variation. For example, while the teacher levitates in the most advanced form of raised lotus pose, we're embarrassed to sit in our simple cross-legged pose while barely crossing our legs.

The wise teacher urges students to honor their bodies and listen to their bodies' wisdom throughout the class. This is how you help a student reach communion with their body.

Comparison with Other Students

Our classroom indoctrination also causes us to compare ourselves with others. My wise teacher Claire also said, "If you struggle to bring yourself into full lotus pose but other students are doing it, wait and ponder: *Who do I have to go home with at the end of every night?*

Me. And who do I have to wake up with every morning? Me." In other words, we might feel compelled to look around the yoga studio, see everyone in full lotus, and feel the pressure to do it, too. But perhaps your knees are telling you, "No way! Don't do it! You'll regret it in the morning." Maybe you ignore your inner voice and do it anyway because you want to look like a badass yogi. In full lotus, you look around the studio so proud of yourself, only to be stuck with a knee brace for the next six weeks.

When teaching, I urge my students not to compare themselves to anyone else. Your journey into a yoga asana practice is between you and yourself. As you look around the room, you have no idea if a student has been doing yoga for five years or five minutes. Some come into yoga with a pilates, gymnastics, or dance background, and others have no fitness routine. The adage, "Comparison is the thief of joy," rings true in this scenario.

After thirty-five years of practicing yoga, I still consider myself a beginner. I'm learning and growing every day. Comparing myself to a twenty-year-old or a one-hundred-year-old balancing vertically, on one hand, would be silly. I have no desire to do that. While it may look cool and make a great Instagram photo, I don't need to look cool in yoga to feel good in my body.

Competition in Yoga

The only way to compete in yoga is to tell yourself you will improve every time you get on the mat.

Students came to my studio for various reasons. Some wanted to touch their toes, others wanted to improve their posture, and some wanted to reverse a medical condition. I had a student whose doctor mentioned she was shrinking, and after two years of practice, she announced that she had grown one inch taller. One student in his mid-forties couldn't sit cross-legged. Little by little, he gained the flexibility to sit cross-legged on the floor without falling over to one side. Another student was able to get off of her blood pressure medications after practicing yoga for a year. One of my consistent goals is to do an additional set of sun salutations without getting tired.

In modern yoga practice, students often create a competitive environment by showing off the latest yoga clothing line and the best yoga gear. Sometimes, it becomes so vanity-driven that the middle-aged mom with her baggy sweats and T-shirt doesn't feel she fits in. Whether you're the yoga fashionista, middle-aged, tired mom, middle-aged fashionista mom, or dad-bod dad, know that the person staring back at you in the mirror is the only competitor you're competing against.

As you enter a stronger union with yourself, you'll know when you're ready to spend five minutes in a headstand. It will feel right and easy. You won't have to force yourself to get into the pose. Furthermore, you won't have to prove to anyone that you can do it to keep up the pace; you'll do it to feel your inner bliss.

Interpreting the Other Yoga Sutras Related to Asana

By lessening the natural tendency for restlessness and by meditating on the infinite, true posture is mastered.

—*Yoga Sutra 2.47*

From this point, dualities cease to disturb the mind.

—*Yoga Sutra 2.48*

I'm not a puppy owner. However, I've observed puppies walking their owners. They are so curious, and some might say, mischievous. Getting a young puppy to do what you want them to do is hard. The puppy will stop every few seconds to sniff a person or a piece of garbage or climb a bike rack. They only let their owner walk a few paces before something else catches their attention. Our minds are like that. They are untrained puppies. Some call it the monkey mind. But I believe puppy energy portrays a much better description of what your mind does daily.

Once you establish a comfortable and steady yoga posture, you feel good. However, your mind might wander to what you're doing after class, what to make for dinner, or why that person next to you didn't put on deodorant. You might also feel anxious about getting out of the posture and into the next one.

In modern times, we're always in a hurry. So, we often feel rushed even when we're not. Yoga class then becomes another thing to check off of our to-do list. When you allow yourself to relax in the here and now, someone might offer you dinner after class, or the smelly person next to you might get a phone call and have to leave early. Let the universe work for you!

While holding your steady and comfortable posture, tell yourself, *I'm doing a great thing for my body. My mind is calmer. I feel my body more fully.* With these mindful thoughts, you'll start to let go of the restlessness. For that reason, I always encourage my students to hold poses with their eyes closed. It provides for a much richer meditative experience. Like the puppy, when you see something, you want to move toward it, even in thought. But if you take away the stimulus, you can focus deeper.

Tension is created when we enter a yoga pose. This is our body's way of sending us messages. Suppose you are practicing *parvatasana*, mountain, or down-dog pose. While adjusting into the pose, your body sends messages: *Your calves are tight. You forgot to stretch after running yesterday. Or you've been sitting too long, and now your lower back feels pain.*

Through yoga asana, you experience the duality of pain and pleasure. At first, the aches and pains come to the surface. But as you release tension and relax, you feel pleasure as your body lets out a sigh of relief. Once you feel that relief, your mind can drift to more pleasant thoughts. Eventually, the pose becomes meditative, and you begin to transcend thought. This is the purpose of asana.

Using Yoga Asana to Detoxify

I'd like to offer a perspective not mentioned in the Yoga Sutras but essential to our modern world. Mat yoga detoxifies the physical body by stimulating the lymphatic system and massaging the internal organs to eliminate toxins. In this section, I will explore using yoga asana to clear your mental, emotional, and energetic bodies.

Logically, the Yoga Sutras don't mention these types of clearing because of the differences between ancient and modern times. Boys in the forest academies of the Himalayas didn't have many distractions. They had to deal with the other students, their guru, weather elements, and perhaps wild beasts, but other than that, the years they spent learning were relatively distraction-free.

Our modern world constantly distracts us. We are indoctrinated by our families, friends, other people, social media, the internet, advertising, and electromagnetic waves from electronic devices. Without knowing it, we constantly absorb the energies of different people and things and carry that energy with us.

For this reason, movement is essential to our well-being. We need movement to keep this energy flowing away from our physical bodies and energetic fields. As we move this energy through and away, we keep prana, our vital life force, moving through us.

Diseases only happen when energy is trapped. It accumulates in an area of the body and forms tension, such as a knot or tumor. When you use physical movement to clear out negative emotions, impressions, and negative energy from others, you keep the pathway clear to your well-being.

Practicing yoga asana for mental well-being is an excellent complement to therapy or other healing modalities. Furthermore, slower-paced practices such as Hatha, Yin, or restorative yoga can allow deeper, relaxed breathing to calm your mind and increase endorphins.

A standing, flowing practice like Vinyasa, Power Yoga, or twelve sets of Sun Salutations (*Surya Namaskar)* can help you move energy more powerfully and detoxify from negative energy you may have taken on from others or the environment.

Living Asana off the Mat

I love living yoga asana off the mat! Most yogis believe they can't practice yoga if they aren't in a yoga class. Nothing can be further from the truth. When you awaken in the morning, sit up, stretch your arms over your head, and sigh loudly as you bring your arms back down, you're practicing asana. You're practicing yoga asana when you hold a shopping cart handle while waiting in line and unconsciously begin to sway from side to side.

Practicing yoga asana off the mat couldn't be easier. All it requires is a constant check-in with your body and adjusting to get into a steady and comfortable posture. For example, when I get out of the shower and begin drying my hair, instead of standing straight, I will lift one leg with my knee on the counter perpendicular to my body as in a pigeon lunge. Or if I'm sitting too long typing on my computer, I will get up, do a half-standing forward fold, and type while bending in half for about five to ten minutes.

Challenge yourself to find five to ten ways to integrate yoga asana into your daily life.

Practicing Asana on the Mat

The best way to practice yoga asana is with present-moment awareness. Pay attention to your body in every moment. As I mentioned, closing your eyes is the best way to tune in. Mindfully move through every part of your body as you hold the pose to relax that part. If you find a particularly tense area, breathe into it. Never force yourself into a pose or variation of a pose that doesn't feel good or provides pain. Discomfort is expected, while pain is not. Pain is a warning.

Focus on gratitude for each body part if you struggle with present-moment awareness. Thanking your body will immediately draw you back to the present. For example, as you move into *pashimottanasana*, seated forward bend, if you can't reach your toes, you might offer, *I am grateful for my toes, feet, insoles, and arches. I am grateful for my hamstrings, my knees, my thighs, my calves, my ankles, and my lower back.* In the few seconds it takes you to repeat these phrases, you will not only snap back to the present but also relax more and forget about your discomfort.

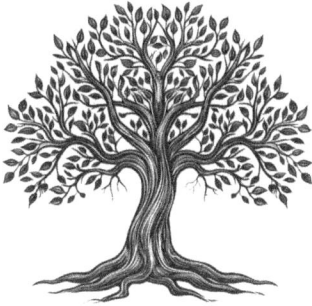

CHAPTER 4

The 4th Limb of Yoga

Pranayama

Breath is therefore called the true sign of life. It is the vital force in everyone that determines how long we are to live. Those who look upon the breath as the Lord's gift shall live to complete the full span of life. —The Taittiriya Upanishad, Part 2, 3-1

B reath is the one thing we can't live without and the one thing we take the most for granted. We can live for some time without water or food, but restrict airflow for five minutes, and we're dead. When a baby is born, she breathes in for the first time, bringing in life without the amniotic fluid of her mother. And when someone expires from this life, the last thing they do is exhale. Breathing is such an autonomic function that we barely give it a thought, and yet it's one of the most powerful tools we can use to bring our body and mind back into balance.

The word prana means "life force." Western words and concepts cannot quite describe this meaning. *Prana* means vital life energy from the standpoint of something vibrant and whole. When a person has strong prana, they glow. Often, someone will say that a pregnant woman is glowing. They see the growing life force within, uncorrupted by poor food, drink, and lifestyle choices. The unborn child resonates strongly with prana, so the mother glows with this energy.

According to Adi Shankara, a Vedic revivalist of the 6th century, we are composed of layers, one of which is *prana maya kosha*, the energy body—people with a strong energy body shine as they walk into a room. A person with weak prana will appear dull and pale. Even if you're new to the concept of prana, you know what it feels like to walk into a room where someone has argued and feel the heavy energy. Or, if you walk into a bar at 2 a.m. surrounded by drunk people, you will feel the sick and desperate energy. Inversely, if you walk into a seminar with an infectious motivational speaker, you'll immediately pick up on the high vibrations. Prana is everywhere in animate and inanimate things.

The Importance of the Fourth Limb of Yoga

The Hatha Yoga Pradipika states, "The purpose of all pranayama practices is to create a perfectly still state in the body so that inhalation and exhalation stop with the cessation of pranic movement." Typically, to get to this state, one must die. However, a trained yogi can momentarily stop the movements of the body and breath to experience this state without dying, which in turn ceases the fluctuations of the mind. This is the entire purpose of yoga, according to Patanjali. Yoga Sutra 1.2 states, *Yoga chitta vritti nirodhah*, which translates to, "Yoga is stilling the fluctuations of the mind."

Practicing yoga asana begins this process; pranayama practice continues it.

The Dynamic Interaction Between the Mind and Breath

Prana is born of the Self. As a man casts a shadow, the Self casts prana into the body at the time of birth so that the mind's desires may be fulfilled. — The Prashna Upanishad 3-3

As a yogi, you are learning to control the mind. With it comes the need to control the breath. Even though holding your breath in a panicked state will cause more stress, holding your breath in a yogic state will increase awareness and bring you to a state of bliss. Intent makes all the difference.

When teaching yoga, I instructed my students to direct their breath into the areas of their bodies that were feeling discomfort. To do this, they would mindfully direct their breath through conscious thought into the parts experiencing pain. That is the effective use of prana. Everyone knows we inhale and exhale through the nose or mouth and into the throat and lungs. Therefore, the trained yogi doesn't take in air through the knees, for example. The intent is to direct the prana.

In the same way, if you sit down to meditate and find that your mind is too active, using simple pranayama techniques such as the 4-count breath or nadi shodhana, alternate nostril breathing, can slow down the breath enough to calm the mind so you can sit still in a pleasant meditation.

The Healing Ways of Pranayama

My oldest yoga student started when she was 92 years old. Dorothy had just come out of the hospital after having had pneumonia. She was weak and needed to be hooked up to an oxygen tank to breathe. Her daughter wanted me to work on breathing techniques to get her off of the external oxygen. Dorothy looked frail as she sat in front of me in her easy chair. Just breathing to stay alive seemed to be a challenge for her. I knew all the yoga breathing techniques but didn't know where to start. I had an hour with Dorothy and was daunted by the challenge.

So I started with *dirgha*, the 3-part belly breath. I taught Dorothy how to breathe from her lower abdomen instead of her upper chest and shoulders. For one hour, we worked on diaphragmatic breathing. The following week, I taught her the ujayaii breath. Each week, I added a new technique. After the first year, Dorothy only needed one oxygen tank daily instead of two. Over three years, Dorothy could do every type of breathing technique and chair yoga. We even added light weights, all because she started with pranayama. That is powerful proof that breath control can heal.

Most people don't know how to breathe correctly, even though they do it all the time. Societal conditioning and improper posture teach us bad habits, and we wind up breathing inefficiently, which leads to many health problems.

When I began teaching pranayama, my students didn't understand how to breathe mindfully. Most would raise their shoulders upon a deep, mindful inhalation, and when I would say, "Expand the belly as you inhale," they usually did the opposite. Societal conditioning tells women, "Suck in your tummy, look thin!" And for men, it's more like, "Stand tall, chest out." Furthermore, suppressing emotions such as crying or exuberant joy causes us to keep our breathing shallow.

Watch a seven-month-old baby breathe. Having recently learned to sit, their posture is tall, and their back is erect. As they inhale, the belly expands, and as they exhale, the belly contracts. That's how we need to breathe!

Proper breathing is necessary for mental clarity, proper brain function, good digestion, and detoxification.

How Breath Control Transforms

In my late 20s, I had a health condition that caused me to start having panic attacks. I had never experienced this inconvenient mind-body reaction, and it scared me.

If you've never had a panic attack, let me explain how it works. It usually starts with a fearful thought. That fearful thought churns with other thoughts, causing your mind to race, your heart rate to increase, your blood pressure to rise, and your breath to become irregular. Many things can happen, such as chest pains and panting.

After having learned that I was having panic attacks, I had to learn how to reverse them. Much of the advice given included various breathing exercises.

Here's how breath regulation works to reverse something like a panic attack.

Since you need to breathe and all systems in your body rely on adequate oxygen to operate efficiently, irregularity of the breath will cause a disruption in your body's rhythms. Furthermore, your thought patterns are directly related to your breathing patterns: the slower the breath, the slower the thoughts. Racing thoughts will always lead to more rapid or irregular breathing patterns.

Think about the last time you received shocking news. Your heart rate likely increased, your blood pressure rose, and you stopped breathing momentarily. In your panic, you held your breath until someone said, "Breathe!" At which point you exhaled deeply.

If something like a panic attack or shocking news can cause your breathing to go haywire, imagine how reversing irregular breathing can lead to calm and well-being.

Prana as the Connection Point to Consciousness

The first and last breath, as the link to life and death, also signifies the link to consciousness. Yoga masters know this and, with this knowledge, strive to master the breath by holding or stopping it with mindfulness. A yogi can lower their heart rate, regulate their pulse, and reach transcendence faster through breath regulation. If you've ever experienced a deep state of meditation, you probably noticed that your breath stopped for a few moments, even as you were coming out of the meditative state. Such power is held in breath control to accelerate higher states of consciousness, including kundalini activation. But as B.K.S. Iyengar states in his book, *The Tree of Yoga*, pranayama is an advanced practice and must be learned only when the yamas, niyamas, and asana are mastered.

Nadis: The Circulatory Channels

Pranayama and asana help awaken the circulatory channels called *nadis*. The 72,000 nadis carry prana throughout the body. While the concept doesn't represent a singular anatomical feature, prana moves through any body part where energy and information are carried. This concept brings to mind veins, arteries, lymph nodes, lungs, the windpipe, colon, urethra, nose, ears, mouth, etc. The central idea in practicing pranayama for detoxification is to keep the nadis clear so that this vital life force can flow freely.

When I learned about the lymphatic system, I was astounded to discover that lymph can't circulate without bodily movements, such as deep breathing or exercise. The lymphatic system is your body's garbage disposal system. So, if you don't move or breathe deeply, your body can't take out the trash. In other words, it can't remove toxins, eliminate old and dying cells, and purge waste products. It's no wonder that a sedentary lifestyle has caused an increase in diseases; the body of a sedentary person is drowning in its muck. When you think about disease versus wellness in that way, doesn't it make you want to get on the mat and do 108 Sun Salutations immediately? Take that garbage out!

According to Tantric philosophy, a parallel body of knowledge to the Vedas, our bodies contain three principal channels: the *Ida*, *Pingala*, and *Shushumna* nadis. The Ida nadi is the left channel representing lunar, feminine, or yin energy. The Pingala nadi is the right channel and represents the sun, masculine, or yang energy. The Shushumna nadi is the central nadi, which aligns with the spinal cord from the base of the spine to the crown of the head. The Ida and Pingala nadis are said to sit dormant, coiled at the base of the spine like two serpents. Through pranayama, asana, and meditation, these "serpents" are awakened and rise in a cris-cross pattern around the Shushumna nadi. At this point, someone might say they're experiencing a kundalini awakening.

Keeping the flow of prana is what makes a person happy, healthy, and whole. And that is why you must breathe with your entire body. A person with open, clean nadis filled with prana often glows, demonstrating perfect health.

The Yoga Sutras Pertaining to Pranayama

Patanjali dedicated five verses to the study of pranayama after having given only three to asana. The importance of mastering the breath cannot be denied. It represents the final physical phase of preparation for meditation.

With a firm posture being attained, the movements of inhalation and exhalation should be controlled. This is pranayama. —Yoga Sutra 2-49

When learning how to breathe mindfully, please keep it simple. The breath in and out should be slow and steady. It helps to count. For example, you can say to yourself, Breathe in for four and breathe out for four. When you feel comfortable, you can increase the count to five, six, seven, and even up to fifteen or sixteen. Later, when you've learned how to steadily and mindfully control the inhalation and exhalation, you can hold your breath as with the practice of alternate nostril breathing, *nadi shodhana*.

The emphasis while breathing may be more on inhalation, exhalation, or on stillness (suspended breath). They can be regulated by space, time, and number and are either long or short. —Yoga Sutra 2-50

Depending on your desired outcome, you might select one practice over another. For example, in *simha pranayama*, lion's breath, the emphasis is on forceful exhalation through your mouth. In the *sitali* or cooling breath, the focus is on a prolonged inhalation through a rolled tongue to cool the body. In *bhastrika*, the bellows breath, you practice with an even tempo between your inhalation and exhalation. And in nadi shodhana, you focus on the count according to a pattern of 1-4-2.

There is a fourth kind of pranayama that occurs during concentration on an internal or external object.
—*Yoga Sutra 2-51*

According to the Yoga Sutras, the first pranayama is inhalation, the second is exhalation, the third is retaining the inhalation or exhalation, and the fourth is when the breath stops through meditation. Previously, I mentioned the breath pausing during deep meditation. This Sutra explains that the focus acquired during meditation causes this to happen without effort. Your breath stops through total surrender.

As a result, the veil over the inner light is destroyed. —
Yoga Sutra 2-52

Your inner light is omnipresent. However, it's been clouded by the fluctuations of the mind. Stressful, fearful, and disturbing thoughts day in and day out continue to cast shadows over your natural light. By quieting your thoughts through pranayama, you let the light peek through the veil. And the more you practice, more light is revealed.

Many people think or say, "I am bad for having terrible thoughts." Or, "I'm a terrible person for not following through (or insert why you think you're terrible)." Contrary to the beliefs of many monotheistic religions, you are not inherently bad. You are intrinsically good. Your inner light is who you are. You've just been trained to cover it up for most of your life.

And the mind becomes fit for concentration. —Yoga Sutra 2-53

This Yoga Sutra previews the sixth limb of yoga, *dharana.*

While I won't address the sixth limb of yoga here, I will talk about the mind. Having taught meditation to hundreds of students, I always warn them of mental disturbances when becoming accustomed to a regular meditation practice.

I first learned to meditate with Dr. Deepak Chopra and his teachers through The Chopra Center in 2007. Although I didn't feel ready at the time, Primordial Sound Meditation was the first course in the curriculum for my Ayurvedic and yoga certificates.

I sat among three hundred participants at The Paradise Point Resort in San Diego, meditating for up to four hours daily and doing yoga classes morning and night. I was thirty-six, living in France with my three kids and two cats, and going through a separation from my husband. While excited for my new path, I feared all the unknowns. On the third day after having learned the mantra meditation practice, I started crying uncontrollably for hours. Even though meditation felt good, the emotional release scared me. The following day, at sunrise yoga, the instructor asked if we had any questions. I raised my hand and asked why I was feeling so emotional. He responded, "Well, that sounds about right. We're about halfway through the week, so it's happening right on time." He explained that when you start to exercise, your body goes through a physical detox. That's why you are more tired and sore than usual. But when you start meditating, you go through an emotional detox. In other words, everything you've suppressed for years and perhaps decades comes out. For someone who hasn't been processing their emotions, letting them out at once can be upsetting. Once I understood what was happening, I could let the feelings come up and release my fears.

In the meditation course I later learned to teach, nothing mentioned this phenomenon. As a teacher, I added it to my course because new students need to be prepared and take precautionary measures. Sometimes, emotions can be sudden and intense. If you can't handle them, you might blame meditation and never meditate again. If a new meditator is aware this might happen, they can be prepared to journal, take it easy, and seek the help of a professional counselor if needed.

In light of this knowledge, you can easily deduct why the Eight Limbs of Yoga are in a particular order. The sixth, seventh, and eighth limbs are about meditation. But if the mind is not yet prepared through the other limbs, it won't be fit for meditation.

Various Types Pranayama and Their Benefits

Modern yoga practice tends to gloss over the importance of pranayama. However, if yoga teachers spent more time teaching students how to properly breathe while holding a yoga pose, students would experience less injury and discomfort and a better state of mind. I don't feel teachers are to blame, but many yoga teacher training programs fail to emphasize pranayama instruction. I had the great fortune of studying with a master teacher who knew its importance and encouraged her trainees to include at least five minutes of pranayama at the beginning of each yoga class.

Here are several types of pranayama and a short description of their benefits.

1. Dirgha: The Three-Part Breath

Dirgha, the full breath, is the first pranayama technique I teach my yoga students. You can practice it while sitting with a tall spine or lying on your back. Dirgha can help you learn to breathe properly throughout your day by correctly using your diaphragm. The three-part breath allows you to take in more oxygen, which calms your body and mind.

To begin, place your hands over your lower abdomen. Relax your shoulders. You will be breathing through your nose with your lips closed. Exhale completely through the nose. Bring your awareness to your lower abdomen below your belly button. Begin your next inhalation by pushing against your hands from the lowest part of your belly. As you inhale, allow your belly to inflate upward toward your navel, mid-belly, and chest. Once you can't take in any more air, exhale slowly through the nose from the chest, mid-belly, navel, and lower abdomen. As you exhale, you will feel your belly contract inward toward your spine. It might feel counterintuitive in the beginning. But the more you practice, the better it will feel.

When teaching the dirgha breath, I instruct my students to imagine their belly as a balloon. On the inhalation, they will imagine inflating the balloon. And on the exhalation, deflating it.

Learning and practicing dirgha is the baseline for all other pranayama techniques.

2. Ujayaii: The Victorious Breath

While I always start a yoga class with the dirgha breath, I continue class with the ujayaii breath. I affectionately call this the Darth Vader breath because it sounds like his breathing. Ujayaii is a great technique in most situations, including holding yoga asanas. We naturally use ujayaii when we are frustrated or upset by exhaling forcefully to blow off steam.

Yet, the ujayaii pranayama is practiced with mindful control.

I teach students ujayaii by having them lift one hand to their mouths and pretend they are holding a pair of eyeglasses. I then instruct them to breathe into these imaginary glasses to create steam to clean them. The sound I make as I blow into my imaginary glasses is a prolonged "Haaaaaa." I point out that fogging their glasses creates steam through heated breath.

Then, I instruct them to close their mouths and exhale the same sound. It will sound like a muffled "ha" sound.

When you practice ujayaii, you breathe in the sound "ha" through your nose with your lips closed and exhale "ha" in the same way. You will use the dirgha breath technique to inflate and deflate the belly. It will take some practice, but ujayaii is an excellent technique that all yoga students should master.

As you practice ujayaii, you are bringing heat to the muscles and calming your nervous system. According to the Hatha Yoga Pradipika, "Ujayaii promotes internalization of the senses and pratyahara" (The fifth limb of yoga).

The only yoga practice in which ujayaii should be avoided is in yin yoga, a cooling practice. It should also not be used if the body is overheating.

3. Nadi Shodhana: Alternate Nostril Breathing

Nadi shodhana is an advanced technique. It balances the hemispheres of the brain and activates the left and right channels, the Ida and Pingala nadis. Before you begin, blow your nose and gently close off one nostril at a time to test which is more open. The nostrils take turns in dominance throughout the day, indicating the dominance of the opposite hemisphere of the brain. At times, both nostrils are open and flowing. This is an ideal time to practice nadi shodhana.

Nadi shodhana brings mental clarity and calms the mind for meditation or sleep.

If you would like a video demonstration of nadi shodhana, here is the link to my YouTube channel with the video entitled Alternate Nostril Breathing | Nadi Shodhana: https://youtu.be/ps8uJkTqrnA.

Begin with a straight spine. Gently place your left hand on your lap with the palm facing up. Bring your right hand up to your face. Lift the index and middle fingers upward to rest on the third eye between your eyebrows. You will alternately block off the right nostril with your thumb and the left nostril with the inside of your bent pinkie finger. At times, you'll hold both nostrils.

The count is multiples of 1-4-2. For example, if you inhale for two counts, you'll hold your breath for eight and exhale for four. You will begin by blocking the right nostril with your thumb, inhaling through the left, holding both, and then exhaling through the right. On the next inhalation, you will block the left nostril as you inhale through the right, block both, and then exhale through the left. You can repeat this cycle as many times as you'd like. Ideally, you will practice for at least two minutes. Your alternate nostril breathing practice will end with the exhalation out of the left nostril.

You will feel a deep sense of calm at the end of your practice. If holding your breath makes you anxious, take time to build up to it. Also, it's best to refrain from nadi shodhana when you have a cold or stuffy nose.

4. Sitali: The Cooling Breath

The sitali breath is great for cooling your body temperature, relieving indigestion, and counteracting the effects of fever and spleen problems. It's a great technique to teach children and those who experience anxiety and panic attacks. I have also taught sitali to my pregnant yoga students to practice during labor and delivery.

To begin, stick your tongue out and roll it inward to create a tube. Some people can't roll their tongues inward, but I've had students successfully learn this technique by pursing their lips with their tongues out. Breathe in through your rolled-up tongue, allowing the air to move in through the hollow space of your tongue tube. You will feel the cooling air move into your body. Then, exhale through the nose. After practicing sitali for about a minute, your body temperature will decrease.

5. Brahmari: The Bee Breath

Brahmari reduces tension, stress, anxiety, and anger. It can also relieve headaches. Its soothing sound brings harmony and happiness. Anyone can practice brahmari. It's a great breathing technique to teach to children.

A simple way to practice brahmari is to inhale through the nose and exhale "Hum" or "Mmmmm" with the mouth closed, mimicking the sound of a bee. Hold the sound for the duration of the breath. If you want to focus on the resonance of brahmari, bring your thumbs up to your ears and press, covering the soft part. Place your two middle fingers over your eyes and let the index finger rest on your eyebrows and your pinky fingers below your cheekbones. Inhale and exhale the brahmari breath for about two minutes. You will feel the intensity of the vibration and will quickly heal from headaches, ear ringing, and fatigue. Brahmari also helps elevate your mood.

6. The Lion's Breath

To continue with the techniques pleasing to children, the lion's breath, Simha pranayama is fun for kids and sometimes embarrassing for adults. That being said, the lion's breath is great for improving your immune system, staving off colds and the flu, relieving tension in the neck and throat, and calming the nervous system.

The simple way to do a lion's breath is to inhale through the nose and exhale the sound "Ha" loudly with your tongue extended outside of your mouth. Continue with the sound for the entire exhalation. To add to the effect, bring your hands up to your shoulders and curve them into claws while doing simha pranayama. Kids totally commit to this, while adults usually burst out in laughter, which is also great for the immune system.

7. Bhastrika: Bellows breath

The bhastrika breath is an advanced and rapid breathing technique with many benefits, including increased energy, improved digestion, toned abs, stimulated internal organs, and increased calmness. However, bhastrika should not be performed by pregnant women and those with hypertension, heart disease, vertigo, and panic and anxiety disorder.

To begin, sit in a comfortable seated position with your eyes closed. (You might want a box of tissues nearby since the forceful exhalation can cause your nose to run.) Inhale deeply through the nose as you extend your abdomen, then in an even tempo, exhale forcefully through the nose, bringing your belly inward toward your spine, and then inhale in the same manner. Do this for one minute, take a break, and start again for two more rounds. If you get light-headed, pause and start when you've caught your breath. Remember that bhastrika, like dirgha, is performed with diaphragmatic breathing, so your shoulders and upper body will remain relaxed.

8. Kapalbhati: Skull-shining breath

Kapalbhati, also known as the "frontal brain cleansing" technique, is similar to the bhastrika breath but with a forceful exhalation and a passive inhalation. It invigorates the entire brain.

Kapalbhati is an advanced technique. Students not accustomed to mindful breathing can become dizzy or light-headed if they move into this practice too quickly. Pregnant women, women who are actively menstruating, people with high or low blood pressure, heart disease, or recent surgeries should not practice kapalbhati.

The benefits of kapalbhati include improved circulation and digestion, better focus, sleep, and stress reduction.

To begin, sit with a tall spine. Place your hands on your lap, palms facing up in *jnana mudra* (the index finger touching the thumb). Inhale for a full belly breath. Then, to the count of fifty, exhale forcefully through the nose with the lips closed. Allow the inhalation to come naturally and passively. Repeat the series three times.

If you feel dizzy during this exercise, stop, return to normal breathing, and begin again.

❧ Living Pranayama off the Mat ❧

Your body already calls you to practice pranayama daily, but as a polite and socially acceptable citizen of your society, you may have learned to suppress this call.

Let's explore some natural bodily expressions of pranayama:

- Yawning loudly
- Sighing with noise
- Morning stretches with deep inhalations and exhalations
- Laughing heartily
- Sneezing
- Breathing heavily or making noise during sex
- Groaning when you hear bad news
- Yelling when you're angry
- Jumping for joy when you're happy
- Squealing with glee
- Singing in the shower or your car

If you're guilty of suppressing your body's natural desire to breathe deeper and release stress or increase endorphins, try a no-holds-barred approach to the above. Obviously, you don't want to sigh loudly when your boss is giving a presentation or yell when it's inappropriate, but allow yourself to experience natural breath regulation daily. You will feel much better for it.

❧ Practicing Pranayama on the Mat ❧

In learning the various forms of pranayama, you will intuitively know which to practice on the mat. Most often, I use the ujayaii breath while holding poses. But I also use the dirgha breath. If you take a kundalini yoga class, you will notice that they use bhastrika while holding a pose to awaken kundalini. As a practitioner of hatha yoga, I find this too intense. Whichever type of yoga you practice, you will find your stride in what is right for you.

Most importantly, it must feel good while you practice. If a breathing technique doesn't resonate with you, change it. I'm a firm believer in listening to your body. Each person is unique and has different needs. Just because your teacher is leading a pranayama technique doesn't mean it's the right one for you. Allow your inner yogi to teach you whether in class or practicing alone.

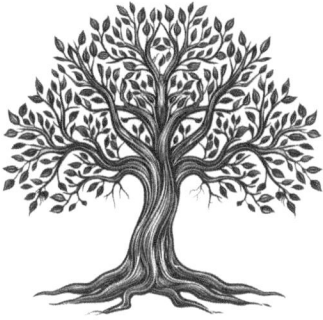

CHAPTER 5

The 5th Limb of Yoga

Pratyahara

*When the senses are withdrawn, the nature of the mind is
calm. Then follows supreme mastery over the senses.*

—*Yoga Sutras 2.54 and 2.55*

Sensory experience rules our human experience.
It's incredible to ponder the value and intensity
of our five senses. Everything we consider an
experience, memory, or imprint comes through one
or more of the five senses.

In 2020 and beyond, those who have lost their sense
of smell or taste from the coronavirus know how trou-
bling losing one or two senses feels. Our sense of smell
protects us from ingesting poisons and gives us pleasure when eating. Furthermore, our sense of smell connects us, on a subtle level, to those we love. As one of

the most primitive senses, your dog or cat understands the intensity as they smell everything to recognize you and their surroundings.

Also, consider those born deaf or blind or those who have lost those senses during their lifetime. They develop an augmentation of the other senses to compensate for the lost one. Since our senses rule our experiences, pratyahara, or "withdrawal of the senses," can seem impossible.

Pratyahara comes from two Sanskrit words, *ahara* meaning "food" and *prati* meaning "away from." The literal sense is to "wean away from." Pratyahara means minimizing sensory input as a preparation for meditation.

Is Pratyahara an Impossible Task?

The most common phrase I hear when talking to clients about learning meditation is, "I can't focus; I have ADD." While some people are diagnosed with Attention Deficit Disorder (ADD) or Attention Deficit and Hyperactive Disorder (ADHD), many say this to mean they can't concentrate. Modern life exacerbates this feeling. When your attention is pulled in many different directions, it can be impossible to keep up.

Advertising, news crawlers, and social media images affect our sense of sight. Our sense of hearing is affected by sirens, car alarms, cell phone pings, and people talking on speakerphone everywhere, even in public restrooms. Our sense of smell is affected by fast-food restaurants piping the scent of fried food outside to lure you in. And our sense of taste is manipulated by companies who want us to become addicted to unhealthy food. Our sense of touch has been affected by the loneliness epidemic of modern times. No wonder many of us feel we can't focus or concentrate.

When I teach meditation, I emphasize the importance of creating the proper environment, especially in the beginning. Quieting the mind can be challenging enough, but if you have to contend with excessive sensory input, it can be nearly impossible.

Several years ago, I was teaching meditation at my yoga studio. My studio was in a tranquil setting, so it was an ideal place to learn meditation. The sliding glass door, which I often kept open during classes, let in the sights and sounds of an adjacent forest and stream. On this particular day, nine students and I meditated for their first time together. After meditation, one woman said it was nearly impossible to meditate with the sound of the angry birds. I laughed out loud as I thought she was referring to the phone app. In reality, she was referring to the birds chirping outdoors. I was surprised she had even heard them, as I had been completely oblivious to the noise. But then I realized, as a new meditator, her sense of hearing had not yet been desensitized. While I had been meditating for nearly a decade, this was her first experience. Hearing is but one of our senses. Now, imagine having to deal with the other four during meditation.

Learning to ignore sensory input is challenging on all levels. Think about it. Meditating makes you hyperaware. Sometimes, you get fixated on what is going on with your body. As you sit, you might be thinking, *Why does my butt hurt?* Or, *Why are my legs falling asleep? Does my heart always beat this loudly? Why is my breathing mimicking my mantra?*

As you learn to withdraw your senses mindfully, you can play with them a little. For example, you can use the annoying sound of the leaf blower as white noise. The challenges that occur as you move your awareness inward become powerful tools for use outside of meditation.

The Five Senses

Control the senses and purify the mind. A pure mind is constantly aware of the Self. Where there is constant awareness of the Self, freedom ends bondage, and joy ends sorrow.— The Chandogya Upanishad 26.2

I've divided this chapter into sections for each of the five senses. Each section contains suggestions to move away from stimulating each of the senses. You can try each exercise as a daily practice or take one at a time for a more profound experience. Consistent practice makes it easier to withdraw each of your senses at the appropriate time. Best of all, you won't be bothered by what others think of you as you engage in this yogic practice because you will learn what is best for you at any given time.

The Sense of Hearing

As demonstrated in my previous example, withdrawing your sense of hearing in meditation or daily life can be challenging. Sounds are all around you. You can either accept or minimize the sounds or ambient noise whenever possible. In modern life, withdrawing the sense of hearing can help you hear your inner thoughts and feelings. We all know how to do this, but we might be reticent.

Many are afraid of total silence. Therefore, you will hear people say they need the background noise of a television, podcast, video, or music as they go about their day. The fear of total silence usually comes from the fear of what is in your mind. In reality, total silence is difficult to obtain. Even if you turn off all devices, you might hear street noise, nature sounds, or the whirring of a refrigerator or heating and cooling system, which can be used to go deeper into meditation.

If the thought of total silence frightens you, it is helpful to explore and understand your fear. Knowing your inner thoughts and feelings can help you transcend your limiting beliefs. With this awareness, you'll have the power to heal your emotional discord.

When I was writing my book *Help! I Think My Loved One Is an Alcoholic: A Survival Guide for Lovers, Family, and Friends,* I interviewed many alcoholics in long-term recovery. One man told the story about how he felt in early sobriety. He explained that during his drinking days, he would drive around with the music on at full volume to drown out his thoughts. Then, one day, after his first few weeks of sobriety, he was driving around with the windows open and music off when he heard the endearing sounds of tiny frogs. He was instantly taken back to childhood memories and the pleasant frog chirps of the spring. He thought, *Wow! Those little frogs have always been there.* He hadn't noticed them for years because he had been trying to stamp out his thoughts and emotions with loud music.

As you ponder the difficulty of sitting or being in silence, explore the following questions.

What are you trying to avoid?

What can't you face within your thoughts?

What is the worst thing that silence can bring you?

What will happen if you're met with your feelings through silence?

Does silence make you feel alone?

If some of your emotions are too intense or unbearable, I always recommend seeing a mental health professional to help you get over the hump. Not everyone can deal with intense emotions by themselves.

It's normal to have general fears. We all have some that are unprocessed. Popular fears include: *I'm not good enough. Will I ever be loved for who I am? What if I'm not successful enough? What if I lose my job? What if a loved one dies?*

When you reach a point in your meditation practice where you can see your disturbing thoughts and emotions, you are ready to heal. This is the upside of seeing your fears and feeling your emotions.

For years, your emotional body has been absorbing experiences that haven't been entirely processed. With our noisy modern lives, when we withdraw the sense of hearing, our emotional body says, "Aha! Now it's my time to speak up!" And speak up, it does. Things you haven't thought of in years tend to creep up on you. Emotions related to past situations you were sure you worked out suddenly come crashing into your reality. At this point, it makes you think two things: one, *I'm going crazy*, and two, *This silence and meditation stuff really doesn't work for me.* Let's explore another example before jumping to conclusions about whether silence is right for you.

If you've ever gone on a diet and tried to wean yourself off of sugar, alcohol, or caffeine, you know how miserable it feels in the first two weeks. You may have had headaches, stomach aches, or feel very fatigued. But you know what to expect if you've tried this more than once. Let's suppose you've cut out caffeine. The first time, you might be surprised at the headaches that occur from withdrawal. The second time, you come to expect it.

In the case of silence and meditation, your emotional body is detoxifying. It's healthy for those unresolved emotions to come up. They've been waiting to be heard. Give them a platform to have a voice. After all, they're a part of you. However, you might be tempted to push them down again. If it's a deeply emotional or sensitive topic, it's okay to ask it to wait to be processed later. Yet it might be wise to have a look if it's something that's been nagging at you for quite some time. I would highly suggest keeping a journal to jot down your feelings and thoughts as they arise. You don't necessarily need to find a solution on the spot. The emotions and thoughts may just want to be heard. But here's the good news: After you've aired your suppressed emotions and thoughts, they tend to taper down with a continued practice of silence. Here's why: as you practice silence, your emotional body detoxes regularly and, as a result, will process emotions more efficiently. You'll no longer keep them bottled up for years. It's liberating to get in touch with what's inside of you. And all of this comes from turning your sense of hearing inward.

Withdrawal of the Sense of Hearing Exercises

The exercises for withdrawing the sense of hearing will differ depending on your chosen activity: meditation, yoga asana, or modern living. However, trying these exercises in every situation will be essential to harnessing the gift of listening from the inside out.

During Meditation

If you're practicing a silent meditation with a mantra, I suggest minimizing your external sound stimuli. Many students ask if they can meditate with music. While listening to meditative music or nature sounds can be helpful in crowded or noisy places, it's best to develop a silent meditation practice. It can be easy to use music or sounds as a crutch. Ideally, you will get used to meditating in a quiet place with minimal noise. Then, as you master drawing your sense of hearing inward, you can try to meditate in a public place and see where your hearing goes. Can you still maintain your focus, or are you easily distracted?

Dr. Deepak Chopra led the group meditation when I first learned to meditate. Before the meditation, Dr. Chopra asked us to silence our phones. Yet, at least one or two phones continued to ring and vibrate during the meditation. For thirty minutes, I could feel my anger well up each time someone's phone rang. The following thoughts bounced around in my head: *Who could be so rude to keep their phone on during a meditation? Why won't they just shut the damn thing off? How selfish can you be to keep a phone buzzing while three hundred people are here to meditate?* After the meditation, Dr. Chopra asked us if we had any questions. I immediately shot up my hand and asked, "Before the next mediation, would you mind emphasizing that everyone must turn off their phones, please?" Dr. Chopra answered calmly, "Why? Can't you meditate with the noise of a phone?" At that time, my answer was clearly "No." However, his comment humbled me. I learned that a true meditator should be able to meditate whenever, wherever, and in any circumstance.

During Yoga Asana

An easy way to withdraw the sense of hearing is to focus on your breath. While we can't always control the noises in a yoga class, we can control our focus. Try to listen to your breath mindfully. This practice will also remind you to breathe deeply in each pose.

In Modern Living

As much as you can, practice sitting in silence. You can turn off all devices in your car or at home when you're alone and learn to appreciate the silence. In social settings, you can practice by speaking less and listening more. It may sound counterintuitive as a "withdrawal of the senses practice" since you're listening. However, your mind will be less chaotic when you sit back, relax, and fully listen to another person. As a quiet observer, you will notice things you've never noticed. You will see the caliber and quality of the conversations around you. You will also start to observe your thoughts.

I often tell the story of another Chopra Center event called Seduction of Silence. Thirty of us practiced silence for three days while the rest of the participants could talk. Our small group attended separate sessions for part of the day; other sessions were integrated into the bigger group. During those three days, I had many unpleasant and surprising experiences.

As the silent observer, not only did my 2010 self get more chatty on the inside, but also more judgmental. I laugh about it now because it was ridiculous, but I began disliking people I didn't know during those three days. It was as if I'd developed X-ray vision and began to see through people via their social masks and ego selves amid the silence. In judging them, I wasn't any better. I felt ashamed. But it also helped me take a closer look at myself and my shortcomings.

Silence tends to improve discernment. When you practice listening and observing, you see things you don't usually see when you're an active participant.

Practice silence whenever you can. Minimize the noise in your life. Speaking in a quieter voice will encourage others to speak more quietly in your presence.

Have you ever met someone who doesn't speak a lot, but when they do, their words are profound? Strive to be that person when practicing pratyahara. Each time I think of this, I'm reminded of the 2012 movie starring Eddie Murphy called *A Thousand Words*. In the film, Murphy's main character is a fast-talker whose life is tied to a magical tree. When he uses a word, a leaf drops from the tree. If he uses 1,000 words, the tree dies, and so does he. As you might imagine, Murphy's character learns to use his words wisely. As you develop on your spiritual path, you start noticing what you say and hear and then decipher if it's meaningful or just noise.

In the beginning, sitting in silence can be pretty unnerving. Do it in small doses if you find too much discomfort. In a short amount of time, you'll find yourself craving silence. And that's when you'll know you're on the right track to pratyahara.

The Sense of Sight

What a beautiful sense! Our sense of sight helps us wonderfully experience the world. When we look into the eyes of someone we love or appreciate a gorgeous sunset, our world seems so much better.

Yet, unfortunately, modern living draws us to less beautiful visuals—for example, disturbing images of tragedy and destruction flash on our screens and devices. Even if tragedy and violence are not a part of our daily lives, we can get sucked into the tragedy of others through images. Many people play violent games with the imagery of pain and death on repeat. Movies, videos, and shows depicting violence are readily available to all at any age. Since our survivalist brain is hard-wired to look for what is wrong, constant images of violence and death can make our bodies and minds believe we're in danger.

The Anxiety Generation

According to The World Health Organization, in 2019, over 301 million people were affected by an anxiety disorder. And only 1 in 4 people receive help for anxiety.[6] Moreover, Millennials are known as the "anxiety generation." The American Psychological Association states that 12% of Millennials have a diagnosed anxiety disorder, which is double the percentage of Boomers diagnosed.[7] One reason Millennials experience more anxiety than older generations is that they were the first generation to grow up with the internet, and social media is one of the culprits of their anxiety. Just as disturbing images can create anxiety, so can images of the seemingly perfect body or life. For Millennials and Zoomers, the reach for perfectionism through social media posts can conjure up feelings of never being enough. Seeing people display posts of a "perfect life" is a constant reminder of how not perfect your life is. Older generations can reason that nothing is perfect. However, younger generations tend to compare themselves to those on social media.

Try A Media Detox for Optimal Health

In the year 2000, when I was healing from cancer and experiencing a lot of anxiety, I read Dr. Andrew Weil's book, 8 Weeks to Optimum Health. One of the exercises in his book was to take a news detox. He recommended refraining from watching any television news whatsoever. Dr. Weil wrote this before internet access to video clips or active advertising across every browser screen. Today, it's difficult to avoid disturbing images, but not impossible.

I have a vivid imagination and a creative mind. Before I refrained from watching the news, I used to have frequent and intense nightmares. I would often wake up in a cold sweat. Additionally, I worried a lot during my waking hours. But after the year 2000, I became very discerning with what I watched. Gradually, I stopped watching TV news altogether. Then, I stopped watching violent movies and shows. I even avoid social media as much as possible. As a result, my sleep and dream patterns improved, and my anxiety dropped significantly.

Perhaps you might be thinking, *I can't live under a rock. Shouldn't I be aware of world events? Tragedy is a part of life.* But as Dr. Wayne Dyer used to say, "You can't get sad enough to make one person feel better. And you can't get sick enough to heal one person." In other words, feeling bad or scared won't help others. Try unplugging from negativity, and someone will notify you if something big happens. They always do. Dr. Dyer also used to say, "If I hear it once, it ceases to be news. News is supposed to be new." Unfortunately, negativity sells, and the more gruesome the image, the higher the ratings or views. When it comes to negativity, you don't have to see it to believe it. If you're inclined to give and help others, do it. But you don't need to pollute your internal environment by ingesting images that aren't helping you. And if violent video games are your thing, it might be worth reevaluating your favorite forms of entertainment as you awaken on your spiritual journey. The energy, rush, and high you get from such games can be mimicked through healthy means such as actively playing in a competitive sport.

Find Beauty in the Present Moment

Mindfully choosing what to look at is the beginning of pratyahara for the sense of sight. Zoom into the present moment and focus on what's in front of you. The power of focus has been lost in modern society. Have you ever watched people in coffee shops? They are often on their smartphones watching a video or browsing social media separately while together. Focusing on what's in front of you has become rare.

With present-moment awareness comes appreciation. You begin to appreciate real-time visuals, whether it's a cup of coffee or a cool car. Appreciating allows you to look for more things that make you happy. In 2018, I moved to Southern California, which had been a lifelong dream. Still, today, as I drive through the streets of Southern Los Angeles County, I look for the beauty of nature that I wasn't able to see before I moved here. I look at the palm trees, the Spanish-style architecture, and, of course, the gorgeous Pacific

Ocean. Even though I see these things daily, I remain in awe every time I see them.

Withdrawal of the Sense of Sight Exercises

Withdrawal of the sense of sight means closing your eyes from time to time to experience your inner world. Additionally, discernment of the visual images that come to you daily allows you to create a better life experience.

During Meditation

The easiest way to experience your internal world during meditation is to close your eyes. It allows you to filter out most external distractions. If you want to meditate with your eyes open, you can focus on a visual mantra called a *yantra*. Typically, these are mandalas comprised of geometric shapes or patterns. You can also use the flickering light of a candle or a beautiful sunset as a visual mantra. However, most of us are not disciplined enough to avoid distractions when meditating with our eyes open, even on a fixed point. Generally, it's best to meditate with your eyes closed.

In Yoga Asana Practice

When you practice yoga with your eyes closed, it's an entirely different experience. You can get in tune with your body on all levels. It's easier to autocorrect your posture with closed eyes, as you can feel when your body is out of alignment.

In Modern Living

You can take measures to minimize disturbing images in your daily life. In addition, you can practice withdrawal of the sense of sight in various scenarios.

For example, when using a weight machine at the gym, I close my eyes to correct my posture or focus on my breathing. I did this once during a personal training session, and the trainer was astonished. Concerned, he asked if I was okay. I told him I was focusing on the task. If you're trying to find a solution to an immediate problem, closing your eyes can help you find the solution quicker.

You can also practice discipline with your sense of sight. Try this: When you see traffic slowed down because of an accident, don't look as you pass by. You'll see how challenging it is. Many people get angry because everyone slows down traffic by rubbernecking, but those who criticize also tend to look. Here is another challenge: Put down your phone for an hour at a time. According to a 2023 article by PC Mag, Americans check their phones, on average, 144 times per day.[8] Practicing visual discipline can help you focus on other tasks. Moreover, a great way to show someone you care is by giving them total visual focus when conversing face-to-face.

The great news is you have a choice. Developing discipline with your sense of sight is like building a muscle: The more you practice it, the stronger it becomes.

The Sense of Smell

I will offer a slightly different explanation of the withdrawal of the sense of smell. Our sense of smell is one of the oldest and most primal senses. Because we are built for survival, our sense of smell is vital because it connects us to our tribe before we can speak. It also helps us recognize where we belong. In addition, it keeps us from poisoning ourselves unless our silly human minds override it. I love what Tony Robbins said about alcohol in his audio program, Get the Edge. While many people poison themselves with alcohol, he used to say, "None of us smelled alcohol for the first time and went, 'Mmmmm yummy!' Most of us said, 'Ew, yuck, bad!' And if you pour alcohol into your dog's bowl instead of water, will he drink it or turn away?" If we listen to our sense of smell instinctually, the scent of something like alcohol will cause us to reject it.

A newborn baby recognizes her mother in the first couple of days of life by her smell. The priming of our most distinct childhood memories comes through smell. My father was from the Middle East and used to cook every day. His sister, my aunt, babysat my sister and me a lot. She spent her days cooking Iraqi food. My childhood brain was primed to think that the scent of Middle Eastern food meant a cozy home life. It wasn't until my early thirties that I stepped into an Indian restaurant. When I did, I was immediately taken back to my aunt's kitchen. I couldn't get enough of those smells and wanted to stay in there forever. I later realized that Iraqi cuisine uses almost the same spices as Indian cuisine. The aroma, spices, and warmth brought me back home. That is the power of the sense of smell.

Using Neuro-Associative Conditioning to Help You Relax

During my yoga and meditation teacher training, I was taught to use neuro-associative conditioning to help induce a state of calm stillness for myself and others using specific scents.

The concept is easy and effective. It's a basic concept taught to first-year psychology students known as Pavlov's dog experiment. Psychologist Ivan Pavlov, the father of modern cognitive behavioral therapy, used a reward system in relation to a signal. He rang a bell to let his dog know food was coming. He would ring the bell, and the dog would be provided with food. He soon noticed that upon ringing the bell, his dog would salivate in anticipation of being fed. Even when Pavlov didn't provide food, the dog would salivate each time he rang the bell.

As in my example with the smell of Indian food, neuro-associative conditioning can effectively take us back to an experience as if we were actually there. The instant I smelled the Indian spices, I was in my aunt's kitchen. I'm sure you can think of some examples where a scent brought you back to a time and place. Have you ever smelled the scent of your first boyfriend or girlfriend's fragrance and felt the emotions of that time? Or have you ever been thrust back into childhood by the smell of a particular thing like an ice skating rink or grass after a rain?

It's incredible how powerful the sense of smell can be to bring up memories. But its power can also be used with certain scents to help you trigger an emotion, change your state, or become more relaxed.

Withdrawal of the Sense of Smell Exercise

Try this exercise to practice pratyahara with your sense of smell.

During Meditation, Yoga Asana, and in Modern Living

Whether on the yoga mat, in meditation, or in modern living, you can "train" yourself to release stressful feelings and thoughts. Choose the fragrance of an incense, candle, essential oil, or perfume that you will use uniquely in your meditation practice. Your goal is to experience the theta and alpha brainwaves of meditation while infusing the smell. The theta and alpha waves ignite a sense of calm stillness, present-moment awareness, and deep relaxation. The meditative state naturally allows these two brainwaves to illuminate in abundance. After 20-30 days of meditation with this unique scent, you can use it in daily living when problem-solving or in a potentially stressful situation. Your brain will remember that this scent was present during theta and alpha states. As a result, your mind and body will immediately return to calm stillness.

The Sense of Taste

When considering pratyahara, withdrawing the sense of taste is an interesting concept that can take many forms. One way to practice this is by fasting or abstaining from certain foods. Another is to mindfully eat less or schedule meals with periods of rest in between.

In our modern world, most people are not in a calorie deficit. Most of the Western World is overfed. According to a World Health Organization (WHO) fact sheet on worldwide obesity, the number has nearly tripled since 1975. In 2022, one out of every eight people was obese, and 2.5 billion adults were overweight.[9]

Humans don't need to eat enormous amounts of food to thrive. Many people have an endless desire to keep their mouths busy by eating or drinking. Ultimately, they aren't enjoying the food or mindful of the taste; they're trying to fill a void or numb pain.

Withdrawal of the sense of taste can mean being selective about the things you put into your mouth. And when you do, enjoying them mindfully.

As a busy mother raising three kids, I didn't always have time to perfect recipes. I often made a new recipe that wouldn't taste that good. So I would eat it, not like it, then eat more of it to be sure. Also, I felt guilty spending so much time, money, and effort making something that tasted terrible, so I punished myself by eating more of it. I know; it makes no sense. I was also raised with the belief that we shouldn't throw away food. In that vein, I became the garbage disposal until I decided my body wasn't a garbage dump.

It's odd what we're taught about food and the sense of taste. When we're little, we might try something we don't like, and our parents urge us to eat it anyway, stating, "You will like it!" Then we grow into adults and can't discern taste. Through yoga, you are relearning how to connect with yourself on every level, and this includes your senses.

Living a yogic lifestyle means eating to live and not living to eat. *The Hatha Yoga Pradipika* states that the successful yogi will have a lean body. This comes through proper discernment and not using the body like a garbage dump, as I did.

Withdrawal of the Sense of Taste Exercises

Try these exercises to use pratyahara for your sense of taste.

During Meditation

To enhance your sense of taste, spend a few minutes meditating with your eyes closed, pointing them first at your nose and then at your tongue.

In Yoga Asana Practice

When I was in yoga teacher training at The Chopra Center, we were taught to wait an hour to ninety minutes after eating before a yoga class. If you don't allow your food to digest, you will be tasting your meal throughout class and might even taste the unpleasantness of your stomach acid.

In Modern Living

Practice mindful eating. In my book, *The Wheel of Healing with Ayurveda: An Easy Guide to a Healthy Lifestyle,* I wrote about the Ayurvedic principle of eating with awareness. Try eating one meal daily in silence, without electronic devices or other distractions. Take the time to taste your food. When I spent a week at Kripalu, a yoga retreat center in Massachusetts, breakfast was the silent meal. At first, it drove me crazy since we also couldn't have electronic devices in the cafeteria. But after the first couple of days, with nothing else to do but eat, I began to enjoy my food and looked forward to the silent meal.

The Sense of Touch

In 2006, I was living in France and retaking yoga classes after a short hiatus. I loved my British yoga teacher's Hatha Yoga classes. So, when she invited me to do a yoga retreat with her, I eagerly agreed. Even though I had been practicing yoga on and off since 1989, I hadn't meditated in silence for more than a minute or two and had only done a handful of guided meditations. During the retreat, my teacher suggested we meditate in silence for ten minutes. Now, here's the tea. We were at a forest retreat center during a cold and damp Spring. Classes were held in a wood cabin with a cement floor. It was hardly my idea of ideal circumstances. But when she suggested meditation, I was eager to learn. She instructed us to close our eyes and observe our breath.

The following describes how my first silent meditation went.

I closed my eyes and began to observe my breathing. At once my mind got very loud.

My God, it's cold in here. It's not only cold; it's freezing. Why are we in a freezing room to do meditation? This is torture. Why did I come here? I thought it was going to be fun. This isn't fun. I'm shivering. And this concrete floor is so hard. My butt hurts. And now my back hurts. Oh, God, why is this taking so long? Okay, back to the breath. Well, I can barely breathe; it's so cold. And now it's raining? Ugh! What a disaster! This floor is killing my back! Why is she okay meditating on the concrete floor? My butt is numb.

My inner dialogue was interrupted by my teacher's voice. "Okay, you can open your eyes." I opened my eyes and asked her, "How long was that?" "Five minutes," she answered.

Five minutes of silent meditation, check, and failed.

Forgetting about the body and withdrawing from the sense of touch is why ancient students were instructed to do yoga asana before meditation. Modern students aren't accustomed to harsh conditions. So if someone says to you, "Sit still and forget about your body," you will likely protest.

Yet, we have the ability to forget about our bodies. We ignore the surfaces or materials it's touching or how it's feeling all the time. Have you ever gone to a party with a friend and declared you had a pounding headache, but when a gorgeous man hit on you, you forgot all about the headache? Or, have you ever been sleepy in class, but when the professor brought up a topic of interest, you perked up?

I had a friend who gave birth seven times naturally using the Bradley Method. She went through labor and delivery with no medication, even though she was induced several times. When I asked her how she did it, she answered, "I go into a deep visualization where I envision the baby's head coming down the birth canal easily as if it's easing its head through a turtleneck sweater." For any woman who has been through labor, you know how painful it is. But my friend didn't feel the pain; she went somewhere else entirely in her visualization, which allowed her to transcend the pain.

Withdrawal of the Sense of Touch Exercises

Try these exercises to withdraw the sense of touch to help shift your focus inward.

During Meditation

As you meditate, when you notice discomfort in your body or physical space, return your awareness to your breath or mantra. It can be challenging as a new meditator to shift your focus, but with practice, you'll become more adept at it. However, if something feels intense, such as pins and needles in your feet due to cutting off your circulation, change positions and then return to your meditation.

In Yoga Asana Practice

It's all about texture, surface, and the right yoga clothes to forget about your body's discomfort. In my studio, I often saw students bothered by their large T-shirts while doing inversions. They spent more time ensuring their shirts didn't lift over their heads than relaxing into the pose. Also, make sure you have a comfortable yoga mat and towels or blankets to accommodate previous knee injuries or pain, for example. Practicing on hardwood or concrete floors without the proper support can bring your focus to the surfaces rather than the alignment and steadiness of your pose. Furthermore, if you're sensitive to the cold or extreme heat, plan accordingly when attending a yoga class where the conditions might have extreme temperatures.

In Modern Living

Unfortunately, modern living deprives us from physical touch. With devices as a barrier to human contact, we need more touch from others and not less. Furthermore, the modern push toward consent and not touching for fear of accusations of sexual harassment or harassment in general makes us starving for physical touch. I agree that some have caused harm through unwanted advances. However, reality states that those are few and far between but made more prominent by media coverage. To feel reconnection to each other and humanity, it's essential to feel the comfort of physical connection. So perhaps, this is one area where withdrawal of the sense of touch might be discouraged for healthy living in modern times.

The fifth limb of yoga denotes the final stage in transcending the human body. Once accomplished, you can focus on transcending the mind through the final three limbs.

Living Pratyahara off the Mat

Having tranquility and clarity of mind is essential off the mat. When we can withdraw our senses and go within, we experience the power of better decision-making. In addition, we learn to trust ourselves more overall. Modern society draws us into a collective mindset likely to be at a lower frequency than our current state. For example, when we follow social media, one person's panic becomes collective, or one person's anger spreads and becomes everyone's anger. For better or for worse, we get sucked into emotions that, at their origin, aren't necessarily ours. Learning how to withdraw your senses throughout your day teaches you to decipher what is yours emotionally and what belongs to others or the collective.

Practicing Pratyahara on the Mat

Distractions are all around us, even in yoga class. Even so, you can practice withdrawing as many senses as possible during your mat practice. A yoga studio or gym class is a perfect way to challenge yourself to be distraction-free.

In modern times, people often get bothered by others invading their senses and expect them to change. For example, I frequently hear women say they're sensitive to scents and will try to talk fellow students into not wearing perfume to class. The self-realized yogi doesn't make anyone else feel responsible for what they feel. Upon self-realization, you know you're responsible for how you feel and perceive the world.

Here are a few suggestions to deactivate your senses during yoga class:

The Sense of Taste:

Many yoga students bring smoothies or coffees to the studio. However, you can drink only water or refrain from drinking during class.

The Sense of Sight:

Try closing your eyes during most poses.

The Senses of Smell and Hearing:

If smells or sounds bother you, try moving beyond them and instead focus on a drishti (focal point).

The Sense of Touch:

If you know you're sensitive to hot temperatures, refrain from taking a heated yoga class. If you tend to be cold, wear the proper attire so you won't be focused on your body's temperature or the texture of the yoga mat, blocks, blankets, or floor.

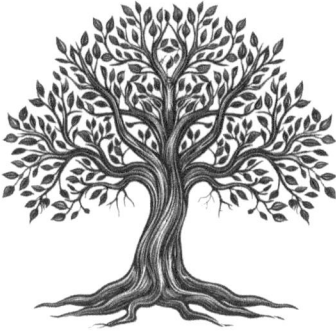

CHAPTER 6

The 6th, 7th & 8th Limbs of Yoga

Dharana, Dhyana, & Samadhi

To be united with the Lord of Love is to be freed from all conditioning. This is the state of self-realization, far beyond the reach of words and thoughts. —The Tejobindu Upanishad

We are now getting to the heart of the Yoga Sutras. The whole practice of yoga leads you here. Your meditation practice will guide you to the point of oneness as you surrender, and the final three limbs of yoga show this process. Since the last three limbs are integrated, it would be fruitless to separate them. As a practitioner of meditation, you come to know this.

Every meditation starts with an area of focus. Ideally, you are sitting or lying down and begin by focusing on your breath, for example. For beginners, this can be a great starting point. But as you advance, you will want something else to focus on, such as white noise (an air conditioner, a fan, etc.), nature sounds (rain falling, the wind, ocean waves), or a mantra. I teach a silent mantra practice, which is how I learned to meditate.

Mantra is a Sanskrit word from two root words: *man*, meaning "mind," and *tra* "instrument." A mantra, therefore, is an instrument of the mind. By repeating a mantra, out loud or silently, you are holding the mind in place so that you, the Self, can move deeper into meditation. The most effective mantras are words with little meaning because the mind likes to take hold of meaning. When I teach mantras, they are comprised of primordial sounds in Sanskrit, which have no meaning for people of most languages. When you repeat your mantra, the mind gets bored and relaxes.

As you continue meditating with your focal point, the uniting aspect of yoga ties together the layers of the Self. In other words, when you release resistance, your body, mind, emotions, soul, and Spirit unite in what Patanjali calls absorption. During this stage, you float in and out of absorption. If you've been meditating for some time, you've experienced this.

Suppose you sit down for meditation. You set the timer for twenty minutes, get comfortable, and begin repeating your mantra. As you focus, you start to feel a rhythm. The mantra may get faster or slower. You find yourself taking deeper breaths as your body re-laxes. Within five minutes, your body and mind begin to settle down. If you hear kids outside shouting and laughing, you notice them and return to your mantra. Another few minutes go by, and you feel yourself get-ting deeper when your doorbell rings. *It's an Amazon delivery,* you think. *Should I get up and get the package? Someone might steal it.* But you decide against it and go back to your mantra. After about ten minutes, you feel completely relaxed. Sometimes, you remember to repeat your mantra; at other times, it floats away. This stage is dhyana, where you move in and out of absorp-tion with your Divine essence. In meditation lingo, some call this "getting into the gap." In other words, you're bridging the gap between your thoughts and merging with your higher self.

As you continue your meditation, you lose all thought, mantra, and conscious awareness. This is sa-madhi, total absorption. Samadhi exists beyond space, time, and causality. You aren't aware you've merged into oneness until you've come out of it. But you will have indications that you've been there, including feel-ings of bliss, serenity, love, and freedom.

This is the culmination of everything you've been working toward in your yoga practice. It's also the en-tire reason for your soul's calling: to return home.

Even though dharana, dhyana, and samadhi don't exist separately, for the sake of this study, let's explore them one by one and then return to this understanding of oneness.

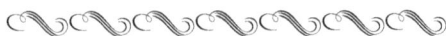

The 6th Limb of Yoga

Dharana: One-Pointed Attention

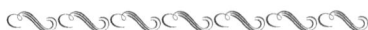

Dharana is concentration, fixing one's full attention on one place, object, or idea at a time.- Yoga Sutra 3.1

In 2018, when I first moved to California, I had left my yoga business and all of my clients. I didn't know how I would make a living until I got established. Thanks to many serendipitous events, I landed a job as a sales associate for Disney Vacation Club at Disneyland. Unfortunately, the job only paid minimum wage for the first four weeks, and any additional income depended on commissions through sales. This was problematic because I had just signed a lease for a $3,330 per-month apartment. During training, we were told that each booking allowed us to earn a commission and that we had to reach the goal of one booking per day. When I did the math, it didn't add up.

To make ends meet, I would need at least three bookings per day, and five would be better. The first week out in the field after training, I booked thirteen appointments and was the number one sales associate that week. Before taking the job, I had virtually no sales experience but a mission to survive. In the first few months, I continued to exceed our sales goals.

The managers started to praise me when I knew the truth: I was flying like a bat out of hell. I was in survival mode. When I told a colleague I wasn't that talented, he revealed something about my success. He said, "You have something the others don't have: extreme focus." He was right. Every day, I set my sights on booking five appointments and would not let up until I came close to my goal. While the others chatted amongst themselves and sat back a little, I talked to as many guests as I could.

The Yoga Sutra uses "concentration" to describe one-pointed attention; I would like to use a better word: focus.

As you begin to feel the integration of your body, mind, soul, and spirit and draw your senses inward, the next step is to focus on a singular object, exterior or interior, to increase the awareness of merging into oneness.

Most people are not good at multitasking. Since the advent of personal electronic devices, multitasking has risen to a new level. We don't seem to have the wherewithal for intense focus unless someone were to drop us off in the desert for a day without devices.

All joking aside, it's challenging to find the space to focus. The Eight Limbs of Yoga practice moves you toward a more disciplined way of being so you can find inner peace. Finding opportunities to introduce one-pointed attention will help you become more prepared to sit for thirty minutes in meditation.

Additionally, mastering the ability to focus on a singular object in meditation, such as a mantra or even the hum of the refrigerator, can help you be more successful in your day-to-day life. People often marvel at the abilities of ultra-successful people when their success is usually due to nothing other than laser focus. At some point, the successful person decided, "I will stop at nothing to make this work." And they did.

We often criticize children for not listening or following orders. However, when left to their own devices, children have an incredible capacity for focus. If you've ever watched a child in an elaborate game of pretend, you know they can get angry if you try to snap them out of it. They understand the necessity of focus in play, while we often do not. Then, we get upset when they can't focus in school. But you can't force focus. It has to come from an internal desire.

I recently adopted a kitten. While most of the time she acts like she can't focus, when it's feeding time, she becomes relentless in her focus. Since she's only twelve weeks old and has a determined personality, she's found a way to get on the kitchen counter when she knows I'm preparing her food. To teach her proper etiquette, I pick her up and put her on the floor. As I turn to pour her food or fork in some wet food, she's back up on the counter. Within a couple of days, she's become faster and faster as her focus on the food gets sharper. The quicker I put her back down, the faster she finds a way back up.

Predator animals, such as cats, have mastered dharana. Take, for example, the eagle. An eagle will wait and focus on its prey. It will only move when it's sure to capture it. An eagle's incredible focus is why I love to do eagle's pose to capture the essence of dharana on the yoga mat. As you twist into a pretzel, you gaze through your hands toward the horizon with the one-pointed attention of the eagle. Once you relax and surrender to the pose, this one-pointed attention feels like bliss.

Living Dharana off the Mat

For one day, try focusing on one thing at a time. For example, when washing the dishes, wash the dishes. When driving, drive without the distractions of a phone call, radio, or podcast. When you're eating, focus on eating. When you're watching a show, watch the show. Immerse yourself in a singular item, experience, person, or task. Notice what kind of resistance emerges throughout your day. Also, notice the pleasantness that occurs as you no longer feel divided in your attention. In your focused attention, the tasks that seemed unpleasant before are now pleasant and even meditative.

Practicing Dharana on the Mat

When practicing dharana on the mat, find a drishti or focal point for each pose. A focal point will help you with meditative absorption.

But if you prefer to close your eyes while holding a pose, your focus can be on your breath, releasing tension from your muscles and joints, or on making autocorrections to relax deeper into your posture.

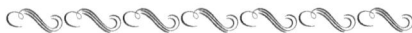

The 7th Limb of Yoga
Dhyana: Absorption

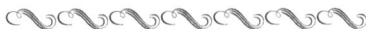

Do or do not. There is no try. —Master Yoda from The Star
Wars Trilogy, Lucas Films

*Meditation absorption is the continuous flow of cognition
toward that object.* —Yoga Sutra 3.2

Focusing on a specific object for a sustained time quiets the mind, calms the ego, and allows your spiritual self to take over. My yoga teacher Claire Diab used to say, "Where your attention goes, energy flows." When your attention is on your thoughts, more thoughts will come. When your attention is on your agenda, fears, or societal conditioning, that is where your mind goes. But when your attention is on your mantra, you ignore the mind, pay no heed to your thoughts, and energy flows to your Higher Being.

This energy makes you pliable rather than rigid and limited. The softer energy allows you to merge with your higher self and divine consciousness, leading you toward samadhi.

The Process of Becoming One

Falling in love is the perfect example of absorption. When you fall in love, you become absorbed with your beloved. The passion is intense in the beginning. You want to spend every waking moment with that person. They're all you can think about. You can't eat and can barely sleep. Thoughts of them flood your mind at every moment. The world stands still when you're with them, and everything else fades into the distance. Time flies, and parting ways feels painful. Your total focus on each other (dharana) coupled with the desire to integrate and become one (dhyana) hastens the process. That person is the object of your desire, and you are theirs. Total absorption with the other feels effortless.

In addition to falling in love, you may have had other experiences that led you to absorption, such as gazing into your newborn's eyes, painting a masterpiece, writing a book, or being in the flow of practicing your favorite sport. They can all make you feel the transcendence of space, time, and causality.

Words to describe this state include flow, divine perfection, synchrony, harmony, oneness, and love.

Attempts to Reach Enlightenment

If you've been on the spiritual journey for some time, you know it's a journey. You may see thousands of people seeking answers and solace from the pain of daily life. In your spiritual search, you might wonder, *Why is this so hard? Or, Why is it taking so long?*

A few months ago, I went to see Amma, the hugging saint. Amma is an enlightened woman who has devoted her life in service to God and humanity. Her mission is to bring love to the world, and she does this in part through her hugs. I received my first hug from

Amma in 2010, and it was life-changing. Afterward, I learned that you can quickly ascend by being in the presence of a person vibrating at the frequency of divine consciousness. Although this was my third time seeing Amma, I was eager to receive my hug.

When it was almost my turn, I sat at the end of the queue. A man in his sixties sat on the adjoining chair and began chatting with me. He recounted his journey to the United States from Australia to live with his guru. He then told stories of meeting many spiritual teachers since 2016. After unloading everything about himself, he asked me if I had a guru. I responded, "Well, Amma is kind of my guru. But then again, I've had many teachers such as Deepak Chopra and Wayne Dyer." My answers didn't satisfy him. "You must have a guru!" He fervently exclaimed. "You will never reach enlightenment!"

After eight years, this man was still seeking a state that evaded him. When he arrived at Amma's embrace, he broke out in wailing sobs. Absorbed in his pain, he was fighting with himself to reach a place of freedom. But he couldn't see that the answers to freedom lie, not in all the gurus he followed, but in the guru within.

Total absorption shouldn't take a long time. Returning to your true nature should feel natural. That said, most people are so conditioned away from their true nature that they think the pathway toward wholeness must be complex. Most protest against the ease of serenity. They say things like, "I could never meditate. I think too many thoughts." Or, "I can never sit still for twenty to thirty minutes. Who has that kind of time?"

Even those who are committed make the process much more complicated than it needs to be.

In our activity-based world, we're accustomed to working hard to reach a goal. To that end, we approach everything in the same manner. We think— *I need to make a list, go step-by-step, get the right clothes, furniture, and items, and then, and only then, will I be ready.* So, you purchase high-end meditation devices to measure brainwaves and the best ergonomic meditation chair. Then you download the latest app of binaural beats to make sure you're ready. After completing these steps, you look at your jam-packed schedule and think, *Well, if I get up earlier and move this appointment around, I should be able to squeeze in fifteen minutes of meditation. I'll start tomorrow.* Do you see how meditation can become a cerebral activity before you even start?

We need to control so much that we don't trust the natural yoking process. But here's what is really happening: you're the one preventing yourself from merging with your spiritual self. And that is why you'll fluctuate between getting in and out of total absorption. Your resistance is the only thing popping you in and out of it.

❧ Living Dhyana off the Mat ☙

At least once per week, go to a place in nature that inspires you. When you reach that space, find an isolated spot and stare off into the distance for twenty minutes. For example, if you're staring at the ocean, allow your attention to focus on the waves as they rise and fall. If it's a tall tree, stare into the high leaves and fix your attention on the fluttering leaves and branches in the wind. Or if you like to lie on the grass while staring up at the clouds, make the moving clouds your point of focus. After twenty minutes, you will feel absorption with your object of attention. And if you still feel separate from it, add another ten minutes. It's blissful to feel at one with nature.

Practicing Dhyana on the Mat

For absorption to occur, you must remain focused for a sustained amount of time. Yin yoga is the perfect mat practice for dhyana. During a yin yoga practice, you hold a pose passively for two to five minutes or longer. Yin is the feminine principle in Taoism. It is cooling, passive, and receiving. Holding a yin yoga pose, such as the supported sleeping swan, allows you to be one with the pose to relax the muscles, ligaments, and fascia. After a few minutes, you may forget you're in the pose as your body surrenders to the posture. While holding poses for several minutes, your thoughts slow down, your mind becomes clear, and your breathing relaxes. Try holding each pose for at least five minutes.

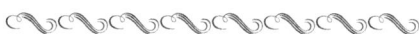

The 8th Limb of Yoga
Samadhi: Integration

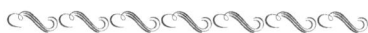

Samadhi is when the object's essential nature shines through, as if devoid of form. —*Yoga Sutra 3-3*

Samadhi occurs when the object becomes formless in the eyes of the beholder. Total integration with Source is when you can't differentiate between you and God. This is God-realization. At this level of realization, you see the oneness in everyone and everything. The artificial barriers separating you from everything else dissolve, and only oneness resides. You cannot force this realization, for it comes with sustained practice. At times, God-realization happens instantaneously. But when you realize you have it, it's gone in a flash. Once you have a cerebral knowing that you've achieved this level, you zip back into individual consciousness. In other words, your brain gets to work. And when it does, you shift back into separateness.

As Dr. Chopra says (and I'm paraphrasing), "We are all a part of the quantum soup of energy and information." Better said, what appears to be separateness is a continuum. Separateness is an illusion. The only reality is oneness.

In the state of samadhi, you move beyond your senses and your body's needs. You transcend your ego, space, time, and causality, and all karma is released simultaneously.

> *He who seems asleep in the waking state, without breathing yet perfectly healthy, is verily liberated.* — The Hatha Yoga Pradipika, Chapter 4, Verse 112.

The Thinning Veil

We are living in a wonderful time for experiencing self-realization. As more people awaken to their spiritual selves, they are paving the way for others to attain enlightenment. For centuries, the road wasn't clear except for a select few who chose to live the life of a yogi or spiritual aspirant. Now, the pathway is widening so that those who seek can find their way faster.

Why Would You Want to Reach Samadhi?

If boundaries are dissolved and you lose your sense of self, why would you want to reach this spiritual state? It sounds absurd. Does it not?

As long as you live in this world and in this dimension of space and time, you will never attain total absorption or integration. For that, you would have to shed your body, in other words, die.

Spiritual seekers, including the Buddha, sought to diminish human suffering. The Buddha even denied his body food, water, and rest to try and transcend its desires. But he realized it's not necessary to try to eliminate the body while you're still alive by punishing it. That only leads to more suffering. Yet through self-realization, where we stand on the fine line of samadhi, we can see the bliss in experiencing this state.

Most people fear death. They run from it and try to push it away through methods to increase life expectancy. Or they forget it altogether and make foolish decisions to abuse this life by drinking, overeating, or taking drugs.

As you mindfully cross the threshold between life and death through meditation, you can taste the sweetness of the other side. In this experience, you come to know that death does not exist. The eternal essence that is you, through your soul, was never born and, therefore, can never die. The loftiness of this state takes you to a bliss that is difficult to experience in normal states. When you've touched it, you'll know. You'll come out of meditation feeling pure joy for no apparent reason. And that is why those who know it come back to meditation again and again.

A Mantra-Based Practice Toward Samadhi

The final stage toward the attainment of samadhi after one-pointed attention (dharana) and concentration or absorption (dhyana) is the mantra. According to *The Hatha Yoga Pradipika* the yogi in samadhi is not affected by mantras, but using a mantra is a means to samadhi.

What this means is that repeating a mantra in meditation is the road to freedom. Mantras are composed of sounds, with "Om" being one of the most powerful sounds. In Primordial Sound Meditation, the type of meditation I teach, a mantra can be composed of three to four sounds. The sound is a vibration or energy. That energy has the power to transform. Meditators have been repeating these sounds for thousands of years to attain samadhi. As you repeat your mantra, you align with all the meditators who came before you using the same sounds. Additionally, when you're taught your mantra, your teacher gives you part of their energy as a *bija* or seed. With this seed, the wisdom gained by your teacher is now yours.

The reason mantras are effective in leading you to samadhi but ineffective in the state of samadhi is because samadhi is oneness. In oneness, nothing is needed; everything just is. If you were to ask God what he (or she) needs, he would answer, "Nothing." God creates for creation's sake and not because he needs something. In oneness, everything is present here and now. You know this when you merge into oneness and transcend duality.

The repetition of a mantra is a flow of energy toward your higher self. That is why preparation for meditation through the first five limbs of yoga is essential. The prepared yogi is ready for a sustained meditation practice to allow the mantra to flow. If you concentrate on the mantra and whether or not it's done properly, you will return to your mind and create more fluctuations or disturbances. But if you release and allow the mantra to float in and out of your awareness, you get closer to merging with the Divine.

Living a Sattvic life

The pathway that led you to samadhi, included the yamas and niyamas, asana, pranayama, and pratyahara. All of these practices prepared you to live a sattvic lifestyle. *Sattva* means purity. A yogi living a sattvic life embodies the qualities of goodness, purity, positivity, truthfulness, serenity, peacefulness, and balance. When you remain in harmony with yourself, you walk in harmony with the world around you.

For example, spending three days eating junk food and binge-watching television will make you feel lazy and lethargic. This is *tamas*, inertia. Your body wants to feel good, so you won't feel in balance with your body.

Or you might do too much hot yoga in the summer. Through your ambitious nature, you power through seven days of hot yoga despite feeling overheated and cranky. This is *rajas*, drive, power, and control. Through this yoga practice, pushing your body to endure harsh conditions to "tough it out" or lose weight can make you lose balance.

The clarity of sattva is total attunement to integration. When integrated with body, mind, soul, and Spirit, you'll know which actions to take when appropriate. You will become a conscious choice-maker who only takes inspired action.

A practiced yogi no longer needs to work so hard to create a beautiful life. Through consistent right-choice making, sattva becomes the most natural choice.

I've abstained from alcohol for many years. I've never had a problem with it, but I've seen how it can destroy lives. For five years, I was in a relationship with an alcoholic and saw the pointless destruction of many lives as a result. I wrote about this in my book *Help! I Think My Loved One Is an Alcoholic: A Survival Guide for Lovers, Family, and Friends.* Even though I choose not to drink alcohol, it's not a popular choice in social circles. I'm often asked if it's challenging to abstain when I'm surrounded by others who drink. Drinking alcohol as a social lubricant is common practice at dinner parties, sporting events, barbecues, fine dining, and most other places where people gather. But it's not difficult for me at all. I care for my body. I want to be clear-minded so I can have fun in any social situation. I've been health-conscious most of my life, and making healthy choices is easy. Furthermore, because I'm mindful of what I put into my body daily, my mind is clearer, allowing me to make better choices.

In the same way, when you choose to meditate daily, your body will crave it. Try it. Practice meditation for thirty minutes twice daily for ninety days straight. After ninety days, if you forget to sit down to meditate, your eyes will close, and you will begin repeating your mantra. Your body and mind will become so accustomed to the blissful feeling of meditation that you won't want to go without it.

Living Samadhi off the Mat

The state of samadhi is not experiential. Yet, through our human perspective, we can mimic the likeness of samadhi by a sense of oneness as expressed in unconditional love. During my yoga teacher training, I learned an exercise called "Having a Namasté Day."

The essence of *namasté* is: *I honor the light in you, which is the same as the light in me, and I know we are one.* When you bow to someone with your hands in prayer posture at your heart center and say, "Namasté," you're acknowledging their soul as one with yours. It's very powerful.

To have a "Namasté Day," for a day, look into every person's eyes, and silently bid them "Namasté." For this to be a spiritual and not ego-based practice, you don't need to place your hands at your heart. You only need to set the intention of honoring their soul as you gaze into their eyes for a moment. You can even silently say, "I honor you. We are one," or, "I love you." To make this effective, choose a busy day where you'll encounter many people. As you go about your day, your interactions will change. They'll become more positive. As you acknowledge oneness with others, they will be more open and loving with you. And even though you aren't doing this exercise to get something in return, you will begin to feel that oneness is your natural state. It will feel good. Your taste of samadhi will be translated into feelings of love.

Practicing Samadhi on the Mat

As you ponder oneness or unity with your body, a holistic approach on the yoga mat can help you transcend limitations. While I'm a strong proponent of listening to your body, I also know that people can live by their limiting beliefs. In my ten years of running a yoga studio and teaching fourteen classes weekly, I heard many excuses about why a student couldn't do this or that.

On the surface, most didn't have apparent bodily limitations, meaning they appeared to be healthy, flexible, and stable. Yet, limiting beliefs can cause a person to stop their bodies from doing what they are able to do.

For example, I had a twenty-four-year-old student who was thin, fit, agile, and appeared healthy overall. Even though she came to yoga, she was convinced that adrenal fatigue prevented her from doing most movements. After several weeks, it appeared that her refusal to move was not due to adrenal fatigue but rather fear of what might occur if she moved. Adrenal fatigue comes from an anxiety disorder where the fight-flight response wears the person out. The more I tried to encourage her that yoga could reverse the effects of adrenal fatigue, the more she dug in her heels, telling me she was too weak to do anything. Her disconnect from her body, coupled with limiting beliefs, created more turmoil in a mental battle she was attempting to win.

Observe your limiting beliefs regarding your body on the mat. For example, if you have declared, "Oh, I can't do lotus pose; I'm too stiff." Or, "I can't touch my toes. I've never been able to touch my toes," connect with your body to see if those statements are true. If you look at your body as a holistic unit, you can mindfully bring your awareness to eventually touch your toes or get into a lotus pose. Like my student who willed her body into limitations through fear, you can love your body into unity and better movement with belief.

On your mat, forget about your injuries and pain. A sharp pain means, "Stop!" But, if you're approaching child's pose and stop yourself saying, "Oh, I have that bum knee. I can't do child's pose." Instead, say, "My body is healthy and whole. I will use a blanket, pillow, block, or bolster to get myself into child's pose because my body works together with me." The idea in samadhi is to transcend the body altogether. Then you can do fun things like levitate. (And, yes, levitation is real.)

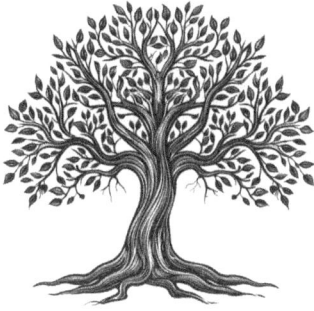

CHAPTER 7

Beyond the Eight Limbs of Yoga

When the five senses are stilled, the mind is stilled, and the intellect is stilled, that is called the highest state by the wise. They say yoga is this complete stillness in which one enters the unitive state, never to become separate again. —The Katha Upanishad, 3-10

By the time we reach the Yoga Sutra verses on samadhi, eighty-seven remain. The study of yoga leads you from separateness to wholeness. And once wholeness is realized, you live through that perspective. Better said, if you can experience God-consciousness, which gives you the knowing that you are a part of everything else, you can attain all knowledge. If you can say from experience, "I am in everything, and everything is in me," nothing can ever be separate from you again.

Chapter three of the Yoga Sutras denotes this phenomenon. In focusing on dharana, dhyana, and samadhi, you gain ultra-focus called *samayama*. Once you've attained samadhi, you can harness the power of various objects. The Yoga Sutras explain that if you focus on the elephant's strength, you will obtain it. The liberated yogi can also harness many powers called *siddhis* or *vibhuti*. Some of these powers include levitation (the lightness of a feather), seeing into past lives, astral projection, or supersonic senses.

Most yoga practitioners won't attain these gifts because they stop at the physical aspects of yoga. Yet, those who have had a spiritual awakening will touch upon certain siddhi powers without knowing how they got them. For example, psychic gifts are among these siddhi powers. The problem is that those who awaken to these powers spontaneously may not know how to use them properly or can't access them at will. The trained yogi has transcended the mind, intellect, and ego. However, the person who has had a spontaneous awakening may still be rooted in fear, karma, and ego desires. If so, using spiritual gifts becomes a burden or may harm others.

When Jesus of Nazareth performed miracles, he had been studying for years. According to the scriptures, he didn't start his ministry until age thirty. Many wonder what he did during those first thirty years. At the time, many spiritual aspirants traveled to India to study under the guidance of gurus. Is it any wonder that Jesus used his hands at his heart in prayer posture, the way people greet each other in India? Jewish people of ancient times didn't greet each other that way. Maybe this means Jesus went to India to study, maybe not. Either way, he spent the first thirty years of his life in preparation. Stories of Jesus fasting in the desert and meditating demonstrated a disciplined life before using his spiritual gifts. He didn't just awaken. He lived awake. His experiential knowledge of samadhi allowed him to heal the sick, turn water into wine, multiply bread and fish, and walk on water. The siddhi powers he lived with were evident to him as a being who lived in oneness.

The fourth chapter of the Yoga Sutras ties together the fruits of liberation. The quest for a spiritual aspirant is to conquer the cycle of death and rebirth and to transcend suffering. The remaining fifty-three Yoga Sutras explain this process.

Desire and karma cause the cycle of life, death, and rebirth. Desires come from latent impressions, either from past lives or from this current one. Karma comes from past lives, and we perform actions in this life that record karmic impressions in each moment. According to the Yoga Sutras, a yogi who has reached samadhi no longer accumulates karma. He has transcended desires and, therefore, lives in freedom.

Here is the reasoning: when you have attained divine consciousness and live in unconditional love, everything you do is for the greater good. But most humans fall back into old patterns because maintaining the state of oneness as divine consciousness is arduous. A handful of teachers, including Jesus, have reached proximity to absolute divine consciousness while still living. They've paved the way for aspirants to see the power within, even though most will dip in and out of it.

So, for the everyday yogi, where does that leave us? If you want to move beyond where you are now, return the practice of the Eight Limbs of Yoga as a study. Meditate twice daily. Explore your limiting beliefs. Practice compassion and humility. Finally, let go of the need to be at any particular place on your journey. You are where you are, and that is where you're supposed to be. As Dr. Deepak Chopra wrote in *The Seven Spiritual Laws of Success*, "I will accept the present moment as it is, and manifest the future through my deepest, most cherished intentions and desires."

Yoga is a lifelong journey. The ancient and profound wisdom of the Yoga Sutras will draw you back time and again because nothing other than the Self is real. The call is you, the real you, guiding you home.

CHAPTER 8

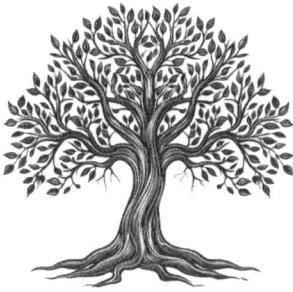

A Special Section for Yoga Teachers

As I gazed out into the recreation room of the assisted living facility, I wondered if I had bitten off more than I could chew. About ten senior citizens stared at me in various forms of mobility, some in wheelchairs, others with walkers, and a couple with full use of their bodies. I had offered my services to expand my yoga teaching, but I wasn't prepared for what I saw. In that first class, I had to modify the poses for various levels with students ranging in age from sixty to ninety. One spunky student stuck out in my struggle to accommodate everyone. She seemed eager and impatient. Her impatience showed me I wasn't moving fast enough since I had to stop to assist everyone else. When I approached her, she asked me if she could do Sun Salutations while she waited. Impressed, I gave her the green light and, at the end, asked her about her yoga experience. "I've been doing yoga for about twenty-five years, and I am ninety years old," She responded. When I picked my jaw up off the ground, I could see it was the power of yoga that kept her so young and fit. At that point, I made the decision to continue my yoga practice for as long as I'm alive.

As teachers, we get much more out of teaching than we give. The yogic lessons taught to us by our students are humbling. Yet most yoga teachers get so caught up in the giving part that they forget to adhere to the yogic principles that led them to teach.

We often forget that yoga students come to us to be led, inspired, and trained. We can only do this if we continue to foster our personal practices and care for ourselves regularly. Even though I meditated daily, exercised, and ate well, I still got burnt out running my yoga studio and teaching fourteen classes weekly. In the end, it was too much for one person to handle.

The difference between yoga gurus from India and modern yoga teachers is that Indian gurus have people feeding and caring for them so they can do what they're good at: teaching. In contrast, most modern yoga teachers have to care for their students and everything else.

Yet, as a yoga teacher, you would be doing a disservice to yourself and your students if you're running on empty or don't have time for your personal practice.

I've created a special section for yoga teachers and teachers in training. Having owned a yoga studio for over ten years, I realize the importance of variety in learning and practicing with yoga students. The more you have to offer, the more your students will grow and evolve with you. For example, I used to run a chakra series for seven weeks during the summer. Students would dress in the chakra color of the week. I would teach the chakra mantras and have poses specific to healing each chakra. In my book, *Chakra Healing for Vibrant Energy: Exploring Your 7 Energy Centers with Mindfulness, Yoga, and Ayurveda*, I describe many of the exercises I used in my chakra series.

Fostering Your Meditation Practice

When I began my studies at the Chopra Center, the first requirement for all programs was to learn Primordial Sound Meditation. It was unclear why this was the first requirement. At the time, my physical yoga practice was more important. After learning and practicing meditation, I realized why. As the Yoga Sutras explains, meditation leads you to oneness with Source. The more you're connected to your higher self, the more you act in accordance with Source energy. In other words, you have more patience, compassion, empathy, and mindful centeredness.

To the best of my knowledge, most yoga teacher training classes don't require a consistent meditation practice as a prerequisite for admission to the program. While meditation has become popular in recent years, I believe it's a safe bet that most people don't know how to meditate without a guided device such as music, video, or audio track with someone else's voice. You'll have an advantage in your personal growth and connection as a teacher if you learn to meditate and practice daily. I teach an online mantra-based meditation class that you can start on demand at this link: *https://www.michellefondinauthor.com/offers/diBP-*

mo2J/checkout. You'll receive your personalized mantra based on your Vedic astrology chart.

You Are Teaching to More Than Physical Bodies

Most yoga teachers outside of very spiritual studios tend to cater to their students' physical bodies first. They fail to recognize that they're teaching individual souls. This is an important delineation to make. And when you make that shift, it will create a world of difference in your students' lives.

As a teacher, you can be self-conscious, unsure of your abilities, or ultra-focused on your lesson plan. When this happens, you can become mechanical and ritualistic in your teaching. You might be focused on teaching the pose properly or having the right transitions. Maybe you're also worried about doing the same poses as the last class. But if you shift your focus to your students and to their well-being on all levels, your teaching will be more natural. You will flow in a way that is appropriate for that class. When you teach holistically, you will notice if your class is tired, stressed, or needs more rigorous action. Souls come together for a reason and purpose, even if no one in the class knows each other. Your job as an intuitively connected yoga teacher is to find that reason. Perhaps the combined souls need a laugh today. And you're the one who provides it for them.

That said, when you're connected to the souls in the room, you're also in tune with their physical bodies. For example, you'll notice if one or two of them are struggling to keep up, and you'll go to them more. You'll also remark if an advanced student is excelling at all poses. So while you're helping the beginners, you can ask that student to demonstrate the next pose. Your class becomes a symbiosis of incredible energy that elevates everyone.

Teaching this way makes it much less about you, your ability to perfect poses, or how seamless your lessons are. In this compassion, you also don't expect everyone to be at the same level. When you're teaching souls instead of bodies, you gain the ability to successfully teach students of various levels in any class.

Leaders Lead

In becoming an Eight Limbs of Yoga-based teacher, you're leading in a different way. You know it's essential to walk your talk. You will work on the Eight Limbs of Yoga practice in your private life and lead with the knowledge of it in your studio. The students who come to you will be attracted to this deeper practice. Then it will be time for you to lead by example.

We are in dire need of teachers who walk their talk. Great leaders lead by example and not only by words. You must remember that yoga is an intuitive practice and that your students will be able to see if you're authentic.

It's possible that you got or are getting your yoga teacher training certificate only to teach in a gym or for some extra income. While that's a worthwhile goal, it's best not to assume that all of your students have the same goals as yours.

If you can learn to teach to the heart of yoga, your physical practice will excel, and the money will come. You can do this even if you're only working in gyms. It's true that most gym managers only care about the numbers or the intensity of the classes for their members. But once the studio door is closed, it's your class. And if you show you're present, connected, and caring, students will flock to your class because you're giving them something more. What's more important is that you are confident in what you're doing and how you teach. If you go in with the intention to connect with the heart of yoga, unity, but are afraid students will complain or won't like it, you won't be effective. However, if you enter with unconditional love and teach intuitively without fear, you will have repeat customers.

When I started teaching prenatal yoga at a hospital, I had never taught that format. I had practiced prenatal yoga during my third pregnancy and had taken an online teacher's class but was afraid I didn't know enough. So I started, sheepishly. And with a weak format, connected with all of my pregnant students on their lives first. I started with introductions and had them talk about their pregnancies. They laughed, cried, and supported one another. Only then did I start the yoga practice. As a result, my classes outgrew every conference room the hospital had. Eventually, I added prenatal yoga as the most popular option to my yoga studio, and I was well-known for the format in my community. However, my success never started with my ability as a yoga teacher. It began with my intuition that pregnant women want to connect with other pregnant women. And in the end, it paid off.

Living the Eight Limbs of Yoga

Living the Eight Limbs of Yoga as a yoga teacher will help you on your life path. Much of yoga teacher training is about theory and technical aspects you might not use. In my seventeen years of teaching yoga, I've never had a student inquire about a specific muscle or muscle group. Most students aren't even interested in the Sanskrit words for poses. They just want to feel better. And when you enter a class feeling great, they want what you have.

The best yoga teachers in my life did two things: one, they practiced the spiritual aspects of yoga, and two, they lived authentically. My three master teachers that come to mind didn't care about looking good and wearing the right clothes. They didn't worry about saying the right things or having the perfect template for teaching; they lived yoga, and it showed.

After thirty-five years of yoga practice the best advice I can give to you is to be your authentic self while teaching. It's the only way you'll be a happy teacher instead of a nervous one. And it's also the way you will have the greatest impact on your students.

And finally, did I mention to meditate?

Wishing you the greatest teaching years of your life. You will gain so much more than you give.

I will meet you in the unified field.

Love,
Michelle

Glossary of Sanskrit Terms

AJNA: The third-eye chakra or sixth chakra located in between the eyebrows.

ANAHATA: The fourth chakra; Anahata translates as "unstruck" or "unhurt."

ANANDA: "Bliss" or "divine joy". One of the highest states of being according to Hinduism, Jainism, and Buddhism.

ASANA: Physical postures; the third limb of yoga.

AYURVEDA: The science of life; the name is derived from the Sanskrit words ayus, meaning "life," and veda, meaning "science or knowledge."

BASTI: Herbal enema using in Ayurvedic practice.

BIJA: Seed; or the seed syllable contained within a mantra.

BRAHMA: God, universal consciousness

BRAHMACHARYA: Celibacy or sexual restraint; the fourth of the yamas in the Yoga Sutras of Patanjali.

CHAKRAS: The energy centers in the body. There are seven main chakras from the base of the spine to the crown of the head.

DHARANA: One-pointed attention or fixed concentration on something internal or external; the sixth limb of yoga.

DHARMA: Translates to "righteous path" or "virtuous duty. An individual's purpose in life.

DHYANA: Meditation; the seventh limb of yoga.

DIRGHA: Also called the three-part or complete breath, a yogic breathing exercise that trains the body to breathe from the diaphragm.

DRISHTI: To view or gaze; in relation to yoga, it means "focal point."

GUNAS: The three fundamental forces or qualities of nature: sattva, rajas, and tamas.

GURU: Teacher means "dispeller of darkness."

GURU DARSHANA: Auspicious sight given to a devotee by an enlightened teacher (guru).

HATHA YOGA: A traditional form of yoga that focuses on yoga postures, breathing techniques, and meditation. Ha means "sun" and tha means "moon" which symbolizes the balance between the physical and spiritual aspects of yoga.

HAHTA YOGA PRADIPIKA: A classic 15th century Sanskrit manual on hatha yoga written by Svatmarama. It is composed of various ancient hatha yoga texts.

IDA NADI: The left subtle channel, which is feminine and lunar in nature.

JNANA MUDRA: Hand gesture of knowledge. It is practiced with the index finger touching the thumb while extending and relaxing the other three fingers.

KARMA: Action or deed. It is also the principle of causality, in which a person's intent in taking an action in the present equals a particular result in the future.

KUNDALINI: Divine female energy that lies latent at the base of the spine.

MANIPURA: The third chakra; Manipura translates as "lustrous gem."

MANTRA: Derived from two Sanskrit words: man, meaning "mind," and tra, meaning "instrument." This instrument of the mind is a sound or series of sounds used to connect body, mind, and spirit.

MOKSHA: Liberation or freedom.

MUDRA: "Sign" or "seal". Symbolic gesture or position of the hands and fingers to enhance the flow of energy.

MULADHARA: The first chakra; Muladhara translates as "root" or "support."

NADI: A subtle circulatory channel running through the body that carries energy and information. The three main nadis are Ida, Pingala, and Shushumna.

NASYA: Method of administering oil or herbalized oil to the nostrils. It is one of the five parts of panchakarma in Ayurveda.

NAULI: A yogic cleansing exercise to strengthen and massage the intestines and internal organs.

NETI: Nasal cleansing

NIYAMAS: Internal observances or duties; the second limb of yoga.

PANCHAKARMA: "Five Actions"; a program of detoxification of the body in Ayurvedic medicine.

PARVATASANA: Mountain pose

PASHIMOTTANASANA: Seated forward bend

PINGALA NADI: The right subtle channel, which is masculine and solar in nature.

PRANA: Vital life energy, or life force.

PRANA MAYA KOSHA: The vital energy, breath, or life force sheath. The energy body.

PRANAYAMA: Yogic breathing techniques; the fourth limb of yoga.

PRATYAHARA: Withdrawal of the senses; the fifth limb of yoga.

PURUSHA: The cosmic Self (soul), cosmic consciousness, or the universal principle; unbounded universal energy that has not yet taken form into prakruti.

RAJAS: Activity, energy, passion, restlessness; one of the three primary qualities of nature in yoga philosophy.

RISHIS: Ancient sages, or seers, from India.

SAHASWARA: The seventh chakra; Sahaswara translates as"thousand-petal lotus."

SAMADHI: An advanced state of meditation, marked by oneness or absorption of the self; the eighth limb of yoga.

SAMAYAMA: The binding of the sixth, seventh, and eighth limbs of yoga: dharana, dhyana, and samadhi. Samayama is when you become the object of your concentration. In Sanskrit, it means "that which binds together."

SATTVA: Purity, one of the three primary qualities of nature (gunas) in yoga philosophy.

SHAKTI: Energy, power, movement, or change; the female principle of divine energy, especially in mythology when referring to a deity.

SHUSHUMNA: The central nadi in the body aligning along the spine; translates as "very gracious" or "kind."

SIDDHI: Supernatural power; realization, attainment.

SUKHA: Happy, good, joyful, delightful, gentle, mild, virtuous

SURYA NAMASKAR: Sun Salutations, a series of yoga poses that coordinates with the breath.

SUTRA: To weave, to thread.

SVADHISTHANA: The second chakra; Svadhisthana translates as "the dwelling place of the self."

SVEDANA: "To perspire" or "to sweat." One of the five Ayurvedic treatments in Panchakarma.

TAMAS: Inertia, lethargy, darkness, or dullness, one of the three primary qualities of nature in yoga philosophy.

TANMANTRAS: Subtle elements. In Ayurveda, refers to the five senses: hearing, touch, taste, sight, and smell.

TANTRA: An ancient set of esoteric texts originally from Hindu or Buddhist tradition dating from the sixth to the thirteenth centuries of the common era; translated as "to weave." tejas: Fire.

TAPAS: "Heat" or "Self-discipline." A yoga practice of disciplinary rituals to purify the body and prepare it for spiritual exercises including fasting, breath control, holding advanced yoga poses, and meditation.

VEDAS: A collection of poems and hymns composed in Sanskrit by people who lived in Northern India in the 2nd century BCE. The word veda translates to "knowledge."

VEDIC ASTROLOGY (JYOTISH): A system of astrology that originated in ancient India and uses the sidereal zodiac instead of the Western tropical zodiac. It is called Jyotish in Sanskrit.

VIBHUTI: Sacred ash from Hindu fire rituals. The ash is applied to the forehead to honor the Lord Shiva. In the Yoga Sutras, vibhuti represents the powers that emanate from total absorption (samadhi), including the power to fly, the power to be invisible, the power to know the great forces of the universe, and the power to move the sun, moon, and stars.

VISHUDDHA: The fifth chakra; Vishuddha translates as "purity."

YAMAS: Moral, ethical, and social guidelines for the practicing yogi; the first limb of yoga, outlined in the first of the Yoga Sutras of Patanjali.

YOGA: Derived from the Sanskrit word yuj, which means "to yoke" or "to join together." In yoga, we join together our mind, body, soul, and spirit.

YOGA SUTRAS OF PATANJALI: The basic philosophical writings of yoga, compiled between 400-600 CE, containing four chapters or books separated into 196 sutras, or aphorisms. It outlines the eight limbs of yoga: yama, niyama, asana, pranayama, pratyahara, dharana, dhyana, samadhi

Bibliography

Chopra, Deepak. *The Seven Spiritual Laws of Success: A Practical Guide to the Fulfillment of Your Dreams.* San Rafael, CA: Amber-Allen Publishing and New World Library, 1994.

Chopra, Deepak. *The Spontaneous Fulfillment of Desire: Harnessing the Infinite Power of Coincidence.* Harmony Books, 2003.

Eawaran, Eknath. *The Dhammapada.* Canada: Nigiri Press, 1987.

Eawaran, Eknath. *The Upanishads.* Canada: Nigiri Press, 1987.

Isherwood, Christopher and Prabhavananda, Swami. *Shankara's Crest-Jewel of Discrimination.* Hollywood, California: Vedanta Press, 1947.

Iyengar, B.K.S. *The Tree of Yoga.* Boston: Shambala Press, 1989.

Iyengar, B.K.S. *Light on Yoga.* New York: Schocken Books, 1966.

Hartranft, Chip. *The Yoga-Sutra of Patanjali: A New Translation with Commentary.* Boston: Shambhala Publications, 2003.

Kriyananda, Swami. *Demystifying Patanjali: The Yoga Sutras.* Nevada City, CA: Crystal Clarity Publishers, 2013.

Muktibodhananda, Swami. *Hatha Yoga Pradipika.* Munger, Bihar, India: Yoga Publications Trust. 1985.

Ruiz, Don Miguel. *The Four Agreements: A Toltec Book of Wisdom*. San Rafael, California: Amber-Allen Publishing, 1997.

Satchidananda, Sri Swami. *The Yoga Sutras of Patanjali*. Buckingham, Virginia: Integral Yoga Publications, 1978.

Endnotes

1 "Yoga Among Adults Age 18 and Older: United States 2022." National Center for Health Statistics. https://www.cdc.gov/nchs/products/databriefs/db501.html. Accessed: October 21, 2024.

2 "New Surgeon General Advisory Raises Alarm about the Devastating Impact of the Epidemic of Loneliness and Isolation in the United States." May 3, 2023. U.S. Department of Health and Human Services. https://public3.pagefreezer.com/browse/HHS.gov/02-01-2024T03:56/https://www.hhs.gov/about/news/2023/05/03/new-surgeon-general-advisory-raises-alarm-about-devastating-impact-epidemic-loneliness-isolation-united-states.html

3 Satchidananda, Sri Swami. *The Yoga Sutras of Patanjali.* Page 122 Buckingham, Virginia: Integral Yoga Publications, 2012

4 "The Larry Bird Work Ethic." https://www.smiconsultancy.com/blog/larry-bird-work-ethic. Accessed November 7, 2024.

5 "Complexity and the Ten-Thousand-Hour Rule." Malcolm Gladwell. *The New Yorker.* August 21, 2013. https://www.newyorker.com/sports/sporting-scene/complexity-and-the-ten-thousand-hour-rule

6 "Anxiety Disorders." World Health Organization. September 27. 2023. https://www.who.int/news-room/factsheets/detail/anxiety-disorders. Accessed: Dec. 9, 2024.

7 "Impact of Mental Health for Millennials." Acenda Integrated Health. https://acendahealth.org/impact-of-mental-health-for-millenials#:~:text=In%20fact%2C%20the%20American%20Psychological,the%20percentage%20of%20boomers%20diagnosed. Accessed: Dec. 9, 2024.

8   "Americans check their phones an alarming number of times per day." Emily Dreibelbis Forlini. PC Mag. May 19, 2023. https://www.pcmag.com/news/americans-check-their-phones-an-alarming-number-of-times-per-day. Accessed: Dec. 11, 2024.

9   "Obesity and Overweight." World Health Organization. March 1, 2024. https://www.who.int/news-room/fact-sheets/detail/obesity-and-overweight. Date accessed: Dec. 11, 2024.

Index

A

Adi Shankara 116
ahimsa 3, 30, 33, 34, 35, 36, 37, 38, 39, 40, 41, 43, 97
Ahimsa 30, 35, 40, 41
Amma 174
Anxiety 148, 207
Aparigraha 62, 63, 64, 65, 67, 68, 72, 73
asana 2, 3, 4, 5, 21, 22, 41, 46, 73, 75, 78, 82, 97, 104, 105,
    107, 110, 111, 112, 113, 117, 121, 122, 123, 144, 159, 181,
    204
Asana 21, 103, 104, 109, 111, 112, 113, 145, 151, 155, 157,
    161
Asteya 47, 51, 53

B

Bhastrika 132
B.K.S. Iyengar 8, 121
Brahma 9, 58, 61
brahmacharya 3, 57, 58, 59, 60
Brahmacharya 54, 55, 61
Brahman 14
Brahmari 131

C

Chopra Center 3, 38, 104, 125, 146, 157, 193
Claire Diab 104, 172

D

dharana 3, 125, 167, 170, 171, 173, 179, 188, 202, 204
dhyana 3, 167, 173, 176, 179, 188, 202, 204

About the Author

Michelle S. Fondin is the author of twelve published books including *The Wheel of Healing with Ayurveda: An Easy Guide to a Healthy Lifestyle* and *Chakra Healing for Vibrant Energy: Exploring Your Seven Energy Centers with Yoga, Mindfulness, and Ayurveda.*

Michelle has been practicing yoga since 1989 and has been a Yoga Alliance Certified yoga teacher since 2008. She holds a Vedic Master Certificate from The Chopra Center including certifications for The Seven Spiritual Laws of Yoga, Primordial Sound Meditation, and The Perfect Health Ayurvedic Lifestyle Course.

She also is an intuitive tarot reader and astrologer. When Michelle isn't writing or recording videos for YouTube, she spends her time at the gym, running, meditating, singing karaoke, and playing with her two cats. Michelle lives in Orange County, California.

Connect with Michelle S. Fondin:

YouTube: @michellefondinauthor

Instagram: @michellesfondin

Website: https://www.michellefondinauthor.com/

Email: michellefondinauthor@gmail.com

Learn Primordial Sound Meditation with Michelle

Start learning on demand with Michelle Fondin's **Immersion Into Meditation Course** based on Deepak Chopra's Primordial Sound Meditation Course. You will learn how to meditate with your personalized mantra in three weeks. With your course fee, you'll receive your mantra in a Zoom call with Michelle. You can also join a thriving community of meditators with group meditations over Zoom twice per month.

Learn more about Immersion Into Meditation on demand: https://www.michellefondinauthor.com/meditation-course-2024-2025

Register for the meditation course: https://www.michellefondinauthor.com/offers/diBPmo2J/checkout

Receive $20 off the course with the promo code **EIGHTLIMBSBOOK** at checkout.

Thank you for reading and supporting this important guide on the Eight Limbs of Yoga!

www.ingramcontent.com/pod-product-compliance
Ingram Content Group UK Ltd.
Pitfield, Milton Keynes, MK11 3LW, UK
UKHW010837090625
6300UKWH00037B/234